ENDORSEMENTS

"Living Beyond Your Chronic Pain is another life resource that 'boomers' like myself will go to again and again for wisdom and counsel from a trusted source, Dr. Joseph Christiano. His book, *Blood Types, Body Types, and You* has provided transformational help to both my husband and me for a number of years and, as a result, he has earned our confidence and respect in all of his research and writing. With his newest book we have the opportunity to consider all of our options, and make well informed decisions regarding pain management. Thank you Dr. Joe for your genuine love and concern for your readers' well-being!"

CARMEN PATE, principal with Alliance Ministries. host of *Truth that Transforms* radio program. Former host of *Point of View* nationally syndicated radio talk show and president of Concerned Women for America.

"Outstanding!!! Joseph Christiano has hit the bulls-eye for pain therapies. If you are in pain and are ready for change, this book is a *must-read*. Dr. Joe offers a *can-do* approach to the full resolution of the pain epidemic."

MARTY MONAHAN DC, NMD

"I cannot think of a more experienced writer to provide this wealth of information for those who suffer in pain. Dr Christiano has firsthand knowledge living with real-life chronic pain and utilizing his scientific mind to find realistic answers from common to cutting-edge technologies. This book is a must-read, if you live with or care for someone in pain."

HELMUT W. MAKOSCH, MC, stem cell scientist

"I want to thank Dr. Joe for tackling the job of helping and educating people with chronic musculoskeletal pain. As a specialist in Regenerative Orthopedics we see such patients every day. The important message is that for many, there may be a simple, safe, non-surgical solution. Today, with the advances of stem cell technology we can now inject a patient's own stem cells and, in many cases, successfully regenerate almost any joint, ligament or tendon in the body. For many, this may address the "root cause" of the pain and restore people to active, pain-free living. I commend Dr. Christiano for taking this important message to the world."

MARK WALTER MD, RegenOrtho.com,
co-founder of Fountain Stem Cell.

"Dr. Joe has taught me invaluable life lessons that I've been able to incorporate into my daily routine. He is an educator, motivator, an inspiration, and a great friend. Dealing with a history of family health issues including being overweight, I now understand that with the proper balance of exercise and the right nutrition the true meaning of what living a healthy life is all about. I would not have been able to accomplish my dreams and be where I am today without his knowledge and guidance. Thank you Dr. Joe, for giving me the tools needed to be the healthiest person I can be. You have changed my life forever! I hope everyone who is in pain will gain the wisdom from all your experiences through this empowering book.

LYNN M. WESLEY, executive producer/
internship coordinator, *Time Warner Cable News*,
24-hour television station, Rochester, New York

"1.5 billion people worldwide suffer from chronic pain, maybe you are one of them. If so, you know how desperately you will seek out any hope of healing or relief. Dr. Joseph Christiano understands. He has given his life to helping people move from hurt to hope, from crushing pain to feeling healthy again and in this newest book, *Living Beyond Your Chronic Pain*, he will give you 8 simple steps to prevent or recover from serious health conditions like osteoporosis, arthritis, joint pain and musculoskeletal conditions. Before you consider invasive surgery try these proven methods to live pain-free. You will be glad you did!"

DWIGHT BAIN, best-selling author, certified life coach, certified executive coach, certified crisis trainer, executive director— The International Christian Coaching Association, nationally certified counselor, founder—The LifeWorks Group

"For over a decade, I have had the blessing of being guided by the wisdom of Dr. Joseph Christiano and have experienced firsthand the fruit of his wisdom as it relates to the health and wellness of my family. As a high-level corporate executive and keynote speaker, who operates on a very fast-paced schedule, my success both in business and life have come through godly wisdom and the alignments of great leaders whom I consider to be my trusted advisers. Dr. Joe has been one of the most prominent voices guiding my family to a place of divine health and wholeness and I would recommend his proven principles to any-one hoping to experience an abundant life of health and wellness. Life's greatest fruit comes at the end of the vine and can only be achieved by those willing to extend themselves beyond what is "normal." Dr. Joe taught my family that what is popular is not always what is BEST. This has been tried and true as it relates to his guidance for our family in turning to alternative options in achieving lasting wellness. We live with physical, emotional, and spiritual peace today and much of that is due to our alignment with Dr. Joe's principles and healing practice."

STACI WALLACE
Sr. Executive of Solavei, Keynote Speaker, Recording Artist, Philanthropist, wife and MOM.

LIVING BEYOND
YOUR
CHRONIC PAIN

LIVING BEYOND
❧ YOUR ❧
CHRONIC PAIN

8 SIMPLE STEPS TO A
PAIN-FREE AND **HEALTHY LIFE**

JOSEPH CHRISTIANO, ND

DESTINY IMAGE® PUBLISHERS, INC.
P.O. Box 310, Shippensburg, PA 17257-0310
"Promoting Inspired Lives."

This book and all other Destiny Image, Revival Press, MercyPlace, Fresh Bread, Destiny Image Fiction, and Treasure House books are available at Christian bookstores and distributors worldwide.

For more information on foreign distributors, call 717-532-3040.
Reach us on the Internet: www.destinyimage.com.

ISBN 13 TP: 978-0-7684-0378-7
ISBN 13 Ebook: 978-0-7684-8430-4

For Worldwide Distribution, Printed in the U.S.A.
1 2 3 4 5 6 7 8 / 18 17 16 15 14

DEDICATION

I dedicate this book to my wife Lori. This book would never have been written if it weren't for her. She carried the emotional load as I struggled through the months and years with chronic pain, failed surgeries, multiple treatments—every step of way. She felt in her heart that I should write a book for those who are hurting and are in chronic pain because I know exactly where they are and how they feel and could relate to them.

How can this man who has been blessed with such a devoted woman let her know her true value and appreciation for all she is to me. As I walk through my healing, I am not alone. I have been strengthened through her encouragement, support, and selfless loving devotion to press on when I didn't think I could go any further.

Not having enough space here for all the accolades you deserve, I lift you above myself to the place of adoration, gratitude and respect that I have for you! Thank you Babe for being *you!* I love you.

ACKNOWLEDGMENTS

I thank my wife Lori who has been with me every step of the way throughout all those painful years. She provided me with comfort and care as well as enduring the challenges that were placed on her like all the nights she slept with me in the ICU room and hospital rooms. I so greatly appreciate her for her loving kindness and support that has made me the blessed man I am today.

I wish to acknowledge some very valuable people who made this "work" a pleasurable experience. There are many behind-the-scenes individuals in which I have not met but want to thank for their involvement in this "work."

I want to thank Ronda Ranalli, Director of Acquisitions and Production, who spearheaded our contract negotiations, follow-up, changes and more changes while making it a smooth uneventful business venture. I want to thank Terri Meckes, Production Project Manager, who is so easy-going and very helpful in directing me with the deadlines, manuscript changes, etc. I also want to thank Mykela Krieg, Communications and Coordination Specialist, who diligently coordinated the layout of the front and back covers, providing the book with the best look and feel possible. And finally Joe Jestus, Chief Matchmaker. From one Joe to another Joe who is responsible for the PR, advertising, and marketing strategies to get this book into the hands of as many people possible, I thank you.

I wish to say "thank you" to Tina Polite & Associates for her tenacity and hard work which eventually brought me to Destiny Image.

There are others who really deserve recognition also. They are those who have helped me find relief from joint pain and damaged joints and cartilage, etc. with cutting-edge technologies and treatments along the way. I want to thank Stem Cell Scientist, Helmut Makosch and Mark Walter, MD. I want to thank Dr. Martin Monahan (my partner at the ReJuv U clinic in Free Port Grand Bahama, Bahamas) from St. Augustine, Florida for the many adjustments in my spine, SI joints and hips. I also want to thank Medical Director Dr. Farshchian, MD who administered the first of many stem cell treatments over the years.

Last but not least, I thank my God and Creator Yahweh for His marvelous design of the human body. How interrelated the human body functions and how He enables man with discoveries and advancements in various treatments and technologies designed to restore the human body back to normal function, only humbles me further of His matchless omnipotence.

CONTENTS

PREFACE

Several reasons why I chose to write this book start with my real-life experience with chronic pain. Firsthand experience works in concert with technology and education when helping others. Second, with a natural, God-given passion for being healthy and having a heart sensitive toward those who are in constant pain, writing this book makes perfect sense. Third, as a naturopathic doctor, I have both experience and academics that can be applied to better serve those suffering with pain. And from an unwavering determination to endure severe levels of pain for months to research remedies, treatments, and cures that may prevent the need for surgery and eliminate the painful process for others, I discovered more healing options to share with people who may have no understanding or awareness of their availability.

My experience is not limited to the competitive individual—I have aided a vast range of people including 40-year-old moms who wanted to get their figures back in shape to top-line executives needing relaxation exercises to cope with stress levels. I have also helped at-risk and obese junior and high school students regain their self-worth and esteem by becoming well-adjusted and physically fit—to various celebrities as I traveled with Planet Hollywood worldwide.

I determined many years ago that the human body was designed and created with such accuracy and pinpoint symmetry that when the body is cared for, it can become very resilient and able to rebound from trauma, sickness, and disease when treated properly. And having been involved in health and fitness both personally and professionally for over 50 years, I have gained a wealth of knowledge in the classroom, in the gym, and on the national stage.

As a competitive bodybuilder and power lifter plus strength coach and consultant for high school and college coaches and students spanning 15 years, my hands-on experience includes application of biomechanics and body works. For example, my expertise eliminated an Olympic skater's crippling pain—who was slated for surgery due to heel bone spurs—simply by adding trace minerals to her daily diet. She avoided surgery and continued skating.

As a professional fitness trainer and coach consultant, I have worked with almost every body type and shape imaginable, as well as a variety of tragic circumstances. Two of many come immediately to mind: I helped a post-op patient regain mobility who had Lou Gehrig's disease and was living on a respirator in a wheelchair, as well as a young female college student regain body strength and functionality whose body was crushed in an automobile accident.

Earning my degree as a naturopathic doctor from Trinity College of Natural Health, I studied, learned, and worked hand in hand with medical doctors who left their traditional "mainstream" medical practices to become part of alternative medicine where they went from treating symptoms to eradicating root causes of health disorders.

My passion is to help people be healthy. I appreciate the responsibility and privilege of caring for people who have been suffering with pain, injury, trauma, or even obesity problems and nurturing them back to normal bodily function and health.

So if you find that I sound off at times in the book about suspicious medical techniques and protocols that mainly target symptoms and not total healing, please understand I am emotional about human life. On the other hand, I hold in high esteem medical specialists schooled and experienced in their particular area of expertise such as cardiologists, heart surgeons, orthopedic surgeons, and the like. I do not disavow the effectiveness of the entire medical community, but I do believe people have the right to know about natural treatment options available to them that address the root causes of disease and conditions.

INTRODUCTION

Imagine living one day without pain! That may seem to be a strange statement, but because you are reading this Introduction, it may not seem strange at all. I bet if asked what level of pain you are experiencing at this very moment, you would be able to tell me in a New York second!

As a naturopathic doctor with years of experience in the health and wellness field as a competitive body builder, power lifter, and fitness coach to numerous Miss USA pageant contestants, I offer proven steps to help you live beyond your chronic pain and enjoy life.

As a professional health and fitness coach who has worked with people like yourself who may be dealing with chronic pain, I know what you are going through. If my assumptions are correct, you are reading this book because you or someone you know is living with chronic pain and want some answers, direction, support, and even hope that there's a light at the end of the dark tunnel of your painful life.

I know how difficult it is to enjoy a full and happy life when suffering from chronic pain. I know what living with chronic pain feels like—from the physical and mental anguish to the cost of medications, treatments, doctor, and clinic visits—not to mention the aggravation of just trying to do normal day-to-day activities. In addition, I know that sometimes it feels like the pain is unique and no one else can understand.

I can absolutely relate to your physical pain, the challenges you face day to day, and the desperation in finding a remedy for ending the crippling nightmare—that is why I wrote this book. The pain I have lived with has ironically provided me an education both academically and through the school of painfully hard knocks—personal experience. All of this has given me a true passion for helping others find the way back to healthy, pain-free living.

YOU ARE NOT ALONE

At times, people who suffer with chronic pain feel like they are all alone with their pain. Yes, they may have the support and love from family members but their struggle is a true reality and a very personal one. From the following statistics, you will see that you are not alone.

A recent market research report indicates that more than "1.5 billion people worldwide suffer from chronic pain" and that "approximately 3-4.5% of the global population suffers from neuropathic pain, with incidence rate increasing in complementary to age."[1]

Please view the following chart. Chronic pain affects more Americans than the pain from diabetes, heart disease, and cancer combined. This chart depicts the number of chronic pain sufferers compared to other major health conditions.

INCIDENCE OF PAIN COMPARED TO MAJOR CONDITIONS		
Condition	**Number of Sufferers**	**Source**
Chronic Pain	116 million Americans	Institute of Medicine of The National Academies[2]
Diabetes	25.8 million Americans (diagnosed and estimated undiagnosed)	American Diabetes Association[3]
Coronary Heart Disease (heart attack and chest pain)	16.3 million Americans	American Heart Association[4]
Stroke	7.0 million Americans	
Cancer	11.9 million Americans	American Cancer Society[5]

This number of people suffering with chronic pain is staggering! If you are one of them, my heart goes out to you as you are experiencing a life that is slowly being reduced to a mere level of survival.

The wisdom shared in this book will help improve your whole life. You will learn:

    a.   Solutions to various painful problems/conditions

    b.   How to identify the root causes of pain and the right remedies to enhance healing

    c.   How to map out your way back to pain-free living

    d.   Answers to your many questions about chronic pain

    e.   How to minimize a myriad of related health problems

    f.   Healthy lifestyle practices specific for you based on your genetics—and much more

Knowing the reality that over 100 million adults are living in the United States with some sort of chronic pain, whether it be pain in the back, hip, knee, neck, shoulder, or other areas of the body tells me there is an entire population of men and women looking for remedies, programs, anything to help them overcome the pain. People in pain want to be able to depend on a reliable healthcare professional, doctor, or specialist who is both knowledgeable in their specific field of expertise but also ethical and conscientious about accurate diagnosis and prognosis of their patient's condition. Unfortunately, there are some in the health field who prescribe unnecessary surgeries for monetary gain, which sometimes incapacitate the patients.

The following list includes a few examples of the various categories of treatments and procedures you will learn about in the following chapters, so *you* can determine your exact condition and then correct it. Some important terms include:

1.   Acupuncture

2.   Myofascial Release Massage (MRM)

3.   Ice or Heat Therapy

4. Anti-inflammatory medications, pain medications, anti-inflammatory injections (Corticosteroid Injections, Epidural Spinal Injections)

5. Adult Stem Cell Treatments

6. PRP Therapy

7. Regenerative Orthopedics (Prolotherapy)

8. Sprains or strains, muscle spasms or tears, etc.

9. All-natural anti-inflammatory supplements, etc.

Because conventional medicine is known for dispensing pain medications as the first line of defense, I want to help you become more informed about the pros and cons of taking pain medications. I am very cautious about the dangers associated with prescription pain medications and the potential for drug overdose, abuse, and addictions. So to help you be more aware of the dangers that are related to prescription pain medications, you will find some very daunting statistics on the topic. I'm a firm believer that being forewarned is being forearmed!

To inspire and encourage you, I have included real-life success stories of people who have left behind the pain and are now living pain-free and healthy because they learned how to naturally improve the quality of their lives by making just one or two very simple dietary and nutritional supplement changes. In addition to charts, glossary of treatments, and explanations, you will be able to identify and map out your treatment choice(s) with better understanding for accurate direction. My entire perspective toward overcoming chronic pain is to implement natural means through nature and science.

As a lifetime advocate and enthusiast of regular exercise, I share the value in proper exercises and stretches that pertain to various areas in your body to support and strengthen the muscles and ligaments that surround and support the joints. It is common fact that when we exercise on a regular basis, we can create a natural healing process that takes the place of drugs and chemicals.

Also included is a regime of food selections that serves two purposes for healing your body from pain and discomfort. Before your body can heal and become pain-free, you must cleanse and detoxify it from toxic metals, drugs, and pollutants, etc. Once that is done, the body will naturally rejuvenate itself so you can enjoy life again.

As people enter the later "boomer" years or become "nesters," their bodies begin to pay back the effects from their previous lifestyles. Whether we were neglectful or abusive by living sedentary lifestyles, suffered sports or automobile injuries, or simply from natural aging, we start feeling and experiencing these effects with each birthday we celebrate. Some people may experience intense or incapacitating pain while others may not, but we all will experience degenerative pain throughout our later years. The goal is to reduce and eliminate these painful effects from continuing further debilitation and poor health by following the simple steps I lay out in the book.

You will learn how to prevent or treat certain inflammatory health conditions such as osteoarthritis, arthritis, rheumatoid arthritis, and fibromyalgia—naturally and without drugs. But even in our best efforts in approaching our injuries and painful conditions with natural remedies, therapies and modalities (body work, stretching, messages or herbal and vitamin supplementation for reducing pain, etc.), there may come the time when we need to use conventional medicine and its procedures.

Though a misunderstood topic, the power of your mind for overcoming any challenge in life is imperative for healing. I will share with you emotional and mental exercises that will help you reduce stress and pain levels—just by the way you breathe. We'll look into developing the ability to overcome pain, reduce your blood pressure, and relax your heart rate which all get out of control when you are in severe pain.

Even in our best educated attempts to overcome the painful challenges that come our way we need the Divine power and healing energy that our heavenly Father Yahweh offers us. In addition to meditation and relaxation exercises that are very positive, I believe in the power that comes through prayer. In our fast-lane world where we almost never have time to chill, we must make prayer part of our healing process.

Also included are *8 Simple Steps to a Pain-Free and Healthy Life* to help you develop a strong body that is vibrant and more resilient to illness, disease, chronic or joint inflammation, etc. These steps are preventative measures for the onset of premature illnesses and diseases as well as painful conditions. These steps also serve as a means for recovering or even reversing your current condition whether enhancing healing treatments or rebounding from surgical procedures.

My motive for writing this book is to encourage you, inform you, and let you know that there is hope. Hope for overcoming emotional and mental battles with those demons taunting you every night and during the early morning hours when everyone else is asleep. Hope in finding a natural remedy or protocol that will bring relief and comfort. Hope in knowing there is a natural way to heal by eating certain foods to prevent joint inflammation and pain. Hope through learning new and unconventional therapies and protocols that you may not have heard of that can be the perfect treatment for your painful condition. Hope that after you have "tried it all" and may require surgery, you will be educated beforehand to know what precise surgery to select to avoid unnecessary surgeries. And hope for overcoming the potentially deadly side effects of taking prescription pain medications and a life of drug abuse and addiction.

Let's walk through your healing together. No more fighting this battle alone. Allow me the opportunity to serve you and provide you with the tools you need to overcome a life of chronic pain.

SECTION I

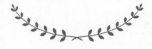

WALKING THROUGH THE HEALING

CHAPTER 1

THE BEST IS YET TO COME

*"One step 'outside the box' can lead
to a better way."* —Dr. Joe

Herniated discs, strained muscles, sore elbow, painful knee joints, lower back pain, epidural injections, X-rays, etc.—it's pure insanity having to understand all the terms, treatments, diagnoses and prognoses, medications, therapies, etc. to treat what ails you. So making the right choice—whether it is surgery, therapy, or lifestyle changes to eliminate your specific pain—is the difference between living a painful and debilitating life or a life that you can fully enjoy.

Before I share with you the many options you have when it comes to living beyond your chronic pain and what treatments await for healing your body, I share the following scenario with you, to see if you can relate to it. If you can, then most likely you have or are living with chronic pain; but if not, I'm sure you know a family member, someone in your circle of friends, a co-worker or relative(s) who can!

> You start off with a painful joint or something like that, and it doesn't go away. You take aspirin or some over-the-counter, anti-inflammatory medication for the pain, but it doesn't go away. You notice that the pain has intensified and started disrupting everything you do. Finding something stronger or

some way to relieve the pain has become a daily issue. It's even disrupting your sleep.

Then you find yourself complaining about the pain everywhere you go and asking family and friends what they think you should do. Some tell you to get an X-ray or MRI (magnetic resonance imaging), and others say to put an ice pack on it, while others tell you to put heat on it. They even suggest that you see a chiropractor or an orthopedic doctor. Perhaps someone has suggested alternative medicine remedies or protocols for healing the body outside of mainstream medicine for alleviating pain. Like most people, going to the doctor is by far your first choice, because by now the pain has become a constant throbbing or burning. It has even invaded your mind to the point where you cannot function normally or live with the excruciating pain any longer.

So you break down and set an appointment with your doctor. Your appointment is at 2 pm and you arrive early with hopes of getting in and out as quickly as possible. First you're handed nearly a dozen forms to fill out, then you have to present your insurance card or some type of medical coverage, and if accepted, you are asked to make a co-pay. This financial expense costs you anywhere from $15 to $70 plus based on if your insurance plan covers it; if it doesn't then it comes out of your pocket. Now you sit in the waiting room patiently listening for your name to be called. After nearly one full hour your name is finally called and you go to a small room to wait. While waiting to see your doctor, a medical assistant or nurse comes in and takes your blood pressure, temperature, and weighs you on the "doctor's scale." By now it is approximately 3:30 pm; almost 1½ hours later, finally the doctor enters the room. He/She immediately starts asking you a series of questions about your complaint(s) and perhaps after a short examination, the doctor goes to the laptop and recommends you take a stronger medication than the over-the-counter drugs you are taking. So a "script" is written for pain medication—take 1 pill four times every day "as needed" for the next 30 days. While at the laptop you are asked if you are taking any other drugs and if you would like them refilled. Why not, you think, there's nothing like a one-stop drug shop. Of course if you were injured you may have been handed a referral script to get an MRI or X-ray to see what the problem is. In either case, your appointment has lasted almost two hours (the actual time with your doctor was just 15 minutes). You see the receptionist to schedule yet another 2-hour appointment; then off to the pharmacy you go.

By the way, if you had an MRI, you experienced something similar to being placed in a giant-size roll of toilet paper. If you weren't traumatized by the fear of being rolled into a tiny space, you may have needed hearing aids after the 30 minutes of listening to some sci-fi screeching and beaming frequency sounds being emitted straight into the cortex of your brain. Of course there is no one there to explain to you what the MRI results showed—they will send the results to your doctor. And you know what that means…another appointment.

Even with the stronger medication, getting around is really becoming difficult. Getting in and out of the car, going up stairs, or just walking from the parking lot to work or to the mall is now has become a painful and somewhat scary experience. Because you hurt so badly and feel a little weaker in your hips, knees, or back, going out became painfully difficult. And to top it off, the pain you experience day in and day out is not only wearing on your body but on your mind as well. In fact, you feel like you have aged about 50 years and are less willing to participate in the fun things you used to like—playing a round of golf, dancing, playing tennis, going bowling.

Maybe after 30, 60, 90, 120 days, you find yourself repeating the entire doctor visit procedure over and over again plus picking up more prescriptions for pain and inflammation. Observing that you are still in pain, your doctor has suggested taking something more powerful; so you are referred to a "pain management group" so another doctor can prescribe stronger medications such as Vicodine, Hydrocodone, Oxycodone, or one of a myriad of other pain medications. Because your condition hasn't improved after taking all the pain medications from your previous doctor, this doctor is licensed to graduate you to taking stronger drugs—narcotics.

Over time you have been led into the medical community's "norm" for living with chronic pain by popping doctor's little helpers—pain meds! But what you may or may not have been told is that narcotics are habit forming—and now a nice person like yourself has become a druggie. After a while, probably many months later, you notice that the dosage and frequency is not relieving the pain as they once did. Now you find yourself at a crossroad. What should you do? Should you increase the dosage yourself until you get relief or make another appointment to see your doctor, hoping for another prescription for a stronger medication? To combat the fears of horrific damage to your body and health as you re-read the side effects of the drugs you're taking, you tell yourself over and over that stomach, liver, kidney damage, and perhaps drug addiction will not happen to you.

If you choose to see your doctor, there is a very good chance that you will be prescribed a stronger dosage, a stronger medication, or even a combination of two or more medications—all of which may provoke deadly results with zero chance of being healed. In fact, the only help your doctor has provided is prescribing some drug(s) to help you **live with** your chronic pain but nothing that could **cure** your pain or reveal the cause of your pain.

At this point in time you may or may not have considered all the horrible side effects and health problems that lie ahead because all you care about is taking something, anything that will take away the pain. So on and on you go living your life with chronic pain, popping doctor's little helpers when the chances are zero of ever being healed by taking medications. And then to add to your dilemma you may experience being chronically toxic, constipation, weight gain, stomach pain and discomfort—and then you realize that you are addicted either psychologically or physiologically or both to the pain meds.

Your pain has been a constant reality for you. Pain medications are not relieving the pain and normal daily functions have become a painful experience. Upon seeing your physician again, he/she is now recommending surgery. (In my opinion, whether you have arthritis, degeneration of connective tissue, or have bone to bone in a particular joint, surgery is the last course of action you want to consider.) Here's what you are now struggling with: after swallowing hundreds and hundreds of pain medications for months and maybe years, the meds have destroyed your stomach, liver, and kidneys—your physical health. Additionally, you are dealing with depression because you realize the pain medications are never going to correct your problem, which means you will always live with chronic pain. Mentally, you think you have lost all hope of recovery and living a normal life again—and now it's time to face going under the knife!

Without a glimmer of hope for living pain-free, you face the ultimate decision whether or not to agree to surgery. Your life has been a downward spiral for months or years. Fear swells up in your mind recalling all the nightmare stories of surgical procedures gone wrong. Your whole life is on hold until you decide whether to live on pain medications, suck up the pain and avoid surgery, or go ahead with surgery and guess about the results. Deep down inside you know there are no guarantees when it comes to surgery. You just have to trust the surgeon with your future—your life. Sure you went out and got a second opinion, read all the literature on the surgical procedure and what to expect post-surgery—the good and the bad. In addition to your mental stress of just the thought of surgery, the fear of never enjoying a normal life, and the constant physical level of pain, you're now confronted with the terrifying and deadly thought of contracting an infection like MERSA or staph that happens more than it should when patients are hospitalized for surgery.

Outcomes of surgeries are mostly unknown; the results can be full recovery and life as the patient once knew it without pain or there may not be any improvement and the patient is in more pain than before. One more thing you may or may not have been told by your surgeon: even if your surgery is successful, your body will immediately start growing scar tissue to protect itself from the trauma of surgery. And when scar tissue grows, it isn't partial to where it grows. So while you experience relief from that sciatic nerve pain or that numbing and burning nerve pain after surgery, scar tissue can eventually grow over the nerve and kind of re-create the crippling chronic pain you thought was gone for good.

WOW! Of course this scenario is just one of many people experience who suffer with chronic pain. Over time their painful life is reduced to a constant routine of doctor appointments, taking multiple medications that only treat symptoms, paying out-of-pocket costs that insurance companies won't cover, experiencing additional health-related problems, continual pain and misery, living a life that is one click above survival at best...until now!

I know exactly what that feels like, and that's why I can help you discover how to live your life beyond the limitations of chronic pain! I will help you map out the best approach to recovery and pain-free living. Let me coach you and educate you about various techniques, remedies, therapies, and healthy lifestyle adjustments to maximize the quality of your life.

CHAPTER 2

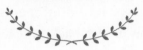

IS LIVING WITH PAIN REALLY LIVING?

*"I couldn't imagine living with all that pain
once I was pain—free!"* —DR. JOE

If you are like most people, through no fault of your own, you probably aren't sure what type of treatment or remedy your specific injury or painful condition requires. Well today is your day! Because today you are going to learn about different types of painful conditions, what to do once you identify the type of pain you are dealing with, what is causing the pain, and better yet, what to do to get relief from your pain.

But before we get into the explanations and definitions and protocols for your pain, I want to briefly share with you why I know so much about pain.

In September 1991, my fiancé, Lori, and I returned home to Florida after spending Labor Day Weekend golfing with her entire family in Jackson, Michigan. Golfing for an entire weekend is nothing out of the ordinary for her family. And because they are exceptional golfers, a lot of pressure was on a "hacker" such as myself at the time. By the time the weekend was over, I had played approximately 108 holes or six rounds of golf. After all the sports, competitive power lifting, bodybuilding, and just nasty falls I had experienced throughout my life, this trip turned out to be the final straw that broke my back, literally.

35

The following weekend, my father and I decided to play a round of golf, 18 holes. As we were rounding the final couple of holes, I felt a really sharp pain in my lower back and legs. This pain wasn't the typical muscle soreness and stiffness after physical activity or muscle overuse, rather something much deeper and much more painful. I realized I had pushed myself over the top the past couple of weekends, so this pain was a warning that something was wrong. When I returned home that afternoon I iced my back on and off for 20 minutes at a time, and continued that treatment for a few days. I also stretched my back and legs muscles to get rid of the lactic acid buildup and soreness, then went on my merry way. I was familiar with various types of muscle pain such as muscle strains, spasms, tears, and overtrained muscles from the years of being a gym rat, so I didn't give it much thought as to the possible severity. It wasn't that big of a deal, I thought.

About one week later as I was getting out of bed on a Saturday morning, I experienced such excruciating pain running down my left leg that it made me collapse to the floor. After being shocked for a moment or two, I tried to stand up again, but I collapsed a second time. This time the pain was so searing and intensely burning that I knew something was seriously wrong with my back. My back and leg couldn't support my body weight, and it became too painful to even lift my left foot off the floor. I actually had to crawl to the phone to call my chiropractor.

After telling him what I was experiencing, he told me to come to his office, immediately! I managed to walk bent over at a 90-degree angle to my car. Driving to his office was an unbearable experience and attempting to get out of the car was beyond imagination. As he watched me enter his office, he started shaking his head and said, "You've really done it this time, didn't you!" I was hurting so badly that I didn't have the strength to tell him off. Obviously, making this painful visit to his office wasn't my first rodeo. I think I helped pay for his mortgage by the number of treatments I had every time I visited his office, particularly throughout my power lifting days.

After his examination he told me there was nothing he could do, and strongly suggested that I stay off my feet, ice my back, and rest. He said he would schedule an MRI on Monday morning. So I did exactly as he told me; I stayed in bed all weekend, what else could I do? While lying in bed all that time, I remembered a woman who saw me walk into his office and said that what I was feeling was equal to or worse than the labor pains she had experienced. She apparently had injured a disc in her lower back and was a mom as well.

Because wedding bells were in the near future, Lori was very concerned about me. She picked me up and drove us that following Monday to a radiology clinic to get an MRI of my back. Sure enough, I had burst the disc in the L-5 joint in my lumbar spine (lower back) with fragments webbed in my spinal cord. My chiropractor agreed with the radiologist that it appeared I needed surgery—emergency back surgery!

I didn't know what to think. I was a high-energy individual living a very physical, competitive life. The biggest scare for bodybuilders, weightlifters, or sports advocates is being told they need emergency back surgery. I thought to myself, *This will put an end to my career, my business, my sport, everything I have done for over 25 years.* I was emotionally terrified! *What about our wedding? What about all the plans we made?* The pain was so overwhelming that I could hardly think. Being the eternal optimist that I am (and petrified of having back surgery), I thought if I just rested my back, iced it, and took good care of it, it would be all right in a week or two. Sorry Charlie, not this time!

After the meeting with the radiologist, my chiropractor made an appointment for me the next day to see a neurosurgeon. I told him there was no way I could handle this pain so he wrote me a prescription for pain medication. This was the first time I had ever taken any kind of pain medication. I felt kind of guilty as if I committed a crime or something. But what could I do, I was incapable of walking upright and unable to cope with the pain—or was I?

MISS AMERICA PAGEANT OR EMERGENCY SURGERY

Other than having back surgery that coming weekend, I had already scheduled a trip to Atlantic City to watch several of my female clients compete in the Miss America Beauty Pageant. I had trained several Miss Florida contestants for the swimsuit portion as well as contestants from several other states. But my current protégé just won the swimsuit competition portion of the Miss Florida Pageant plus the crown. We worked together for most of the year in preparation for this big event.

The next day I kept my appointment with the neurosurgeon. After examining my MRI, he said, "You need emergency surgery, and you need it now!" I asked him how serious it was and he said, "If you don't get it done immediately, you may have permanent nerve damage that will leave you with a floppy left foot for life." I had already started losing dorsiflexion in my left foot, which is the ability to lift your toes off the ground as when you walk or tap your toes on the ground. I asked him what could I expect from having the surgery, and he said one of three things will happen: I would recover completely and go back to normal living, I would partially recover to a portion of normal living, or I could be paralyzed for the rest of my life. After a huge gulp, I told him I needed a day to think it over and pray about it. He said, "Don't waste too much time!"

All that night a million thoughts were running through my mind. I had so many huge decisions to make that included marriage, my career, and walking or not walking—not necessarily in that particular order. But the most immediate one that had a lot to do with growing my fitness business was going to Atlantic City to attend the Miss America Pageant and be there for my Miss Florida client who had a good chance of winning the swimsuit competition. Our local news would be there, national news and TV was there, plus I already had several swimsuit winners in the Miss America and Miss USA pageants; so being there that coming weekend would be a huge opportunity to get national exposure for my fitness business. This weekend trip would be a good business move.

The next morning I decided not to take the pain medications. I wanted to see if I could manage my day without them; if I could, I was heading to Atlantic City. If not, I'd have the surgery. Well, by the middle of lunch I found myself on the floor again in excruciating pain. The obvious writing was on the wall. I had no other option but to go under the knife, the very thing I dreaded and the very thing I thought would ruin my physical life as I knew it. But what could I do? After work, Lori and I talked about it over and over, we prayed about it, but the pain was so great that I had no choice.

So that Saturday morning, instead of being in Atlantic City encouraging my clients and my Miss Florida protégé with last minute tips before the evening show, I was being prepped for emergency back surgery.

RECOVERY

After the two-hour surgery and half-hour recovery, I started wiggling and moving my toes and feet to check and see if they were still functioning normally. They were—what a huge mental relief. Just before being wheeled out of the recovery room to my room, a few nurses started asking me how to reshape their bodies like the pageant contestants. I spent the whole day sleeping on and off, but by early evening I had a lot of energy and didn't need any pain meds. Lori and my folks were there, so we decided to watch the Miss America Beauty Pageant.

The contestants went through their normal portions of competition, and when the final top ten were called out, Miss Florida was one of them! She also won the swimsuit portion. I was almost jumping out of the bed. Then Bert Parks announced the final two contestants, one being Miss Florida. Who do you suppose won the whole enchilada? Not only did my Miss Florida protégé, LeeAnn Cornet, win the swimsuit competition, she also won the entire pageant and was crowned the new Miss America. Go figure!

The next morning I got out of bed and felt okay. I was a little weak but no big deal. Standing up for the first time since my surgery, I just realized I had *no* pain! I was so excited. I was ready to go home. I cleaned up the area around my bed, got dressed, and sat in a chair waiting for my surgeon to visit. When he arrived, he asked, "What are you doing out of bed?" I told him I felt great and got dressed to go home. "Home?" he said, "My back surgery patients generally need two to three weeks of treatment and post-surgery therapy." I asked what I needed to do to rehabilitate my back because I could do it myself at home. He looked at me and said, "Yeah, you probably know more about that stuff than I do anyway." So I was released from the hospital only 23 hours after surgery.

MAKING THE COMEBACK

At home I started self therapy. I couldn't help but remember what the surgeon had said were the likely results after surgery. Thankfully, my pain was gone. I could walk upright, and everything seemed to be normal, so I was bent on going to the mountain one more time. (Going to the mountain is a favorite expression when I have to start all over in a project, goal, or start something anew.)

Oh, I forgot to mention that Lori and I waited an entire year after canceling our wedding plans due to the back surgery. So the following year we went to Jamaica for a two-week wedding and honeymoon. After dating six and a half years, getting married was a hand and glove experience. Needless to say, we danced our nights away while listening to steel drums and Reggae music. Now, it was time to build our lives and the business together. We had great plans for the future.

Life was perfect, even though I still had a little twinge of pain in my lower back.

CHAPTER 3

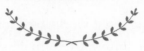

Try Everything Else before Considering Surgery

*"Options! Options! Options! Try them, you
just might find the right one!"*—Dr. Joe

Being married for nearly 15 years, it had also been that long since back surgery. And in my case, the emergency surgery was a success, for I had returned to doing just about everything I did before, from strength training to snow skiing to golfing, taking long evening walks with Lori, even bowling. Fifteen years after surgery was also the same time Lori and I moved into our new home, a successful project with no major pain—until weeks afterward.

After the move was over and months later, that lower back pain demon began to show its ugly face again. The level of pain was a 7 or 8 and sometimes a 10 plus, on a day-to-day basis. It started to overwhelm me as it began to affect my daily activities, business, travel, training, and everything else. I thought, *Please, not again!* If you have had back surgery or musculoskeletal surgery, you know exactly what I mean.

Pain is a natural indicator telling you something is wrong. A word to the wise: try every possible means of natural therapeutic protocols and remedies under the sun before entertaining the prospects of surgery, because of the possible negative outcome.

THE TIP OF THE ICEBERG

The key to discovering what works best for your condition is to listen to your body, try the simplest treatment(s), and be in tune to how your body responds. Based on how you feel determines if you stay with that particular treatment or try something more advanced. Because my condition worsened and wasn't improving, I agreed to weekly chiropractic treatments that included various treatments and protocols from gentle massage therapy to muscle testing to factoring in mental and emotion stressors. We had sit-down consultations when we discussed lifestyle practices and attitudes about living with pain. I recall her soft and nurturing voice saying, *"When dealing with pain, it is not about how much pain we can endure for a lifetime but finding a way to rid our life of pain."*

I had endured lower back pain for much of my life from all the years my body took a pounding, especially from contact sports, competitive power lifting, and body building; with that came a high pain threshold. But we know where that got me—emergency back surgery. But after enjoying pain-free living for nearly 15 years, I wasn't about to cave to the pain. The constant searing nerve pain I was feeling again was all it took for me to start a thorough search for the correct treatment and modalities I needed. It was time to try everything under the sun before considering back surgery. Maybe my chiropractor was correct about finding a way to rid myself of pain.

A BLESSING OR A CURSE

Change does not come easy and relearning not to endure chronic pain wasn't an overnight change for me either. I recall the time my physical therapist came to my house to do deep muscle tissue massage on my shoulder after I had re-injured it. Sometimes when we sustain an injury or re-injure ourselves and don't allow it to properly heal, the muscle can form scar tissue (scar tissue will also form after having a surgery). Scar tissue develops where there was a tear or strain in the muscle fiber. The scar tissue becomes very hard and will not allow the muscle to stretch properly throughout the ROM (range of motion) of an adjacent joint, making movement very painful. Trying to move the shoulder or arm is a very painful experience, which was my case.

The therapist said to use an ice pack on it until he arrived. Normally I placed a towel or some type of thick cloth between the ice pack and my skin to avoid an ice burn. *Ice pack therapy is the best first-line therapy to use immediately after you sustain an injury or re-injure yourself because it reduces the inflammation or swollen tissue in the area.* To be honest I couldn't feel the freezing effect of the ice pack, so I removed the cloth and placed the ice pack against my bare shoulder. Sure it was uncomfortable but it wasn't all that painful. By the time the therapist arrived I had caused an ice burn to my skin tissue. When he saw the dark red discoloration of my skin, he asked, "Didn't you feel it burning your skin?" I told him I felt it burning but it wasn't too painful.

I have to admit that living with and enduring chronic pain resulted in a high pain threshold for so many years that it created a domino effect causing other health issues. Over time I was experiencing neuropathy or nerve damage and nerve pain. This occurs when a nerve is pinched by swollen muscle tissue or a vertebra disc in the spinal cord. By this point I had already lost most of the feeling in my left thigh plus feelings in two toes on my right foot. Even the pad on my foot was numb to the point that it felt like I was stepping on a small mound of some sort when the pad of my foot would touch the floor. The nerve signals or messages from the brain that traveled down the spinal cord and through my lower limbs were being affected. Now I was dealing with chronic pain and neuropathy.

If you suffer with chronic pain you know it affects other areas of your body and health as well. Here's another example of the domino effect it had on my health. One evening Lori and I were out for dinner when all of a sudden I had a gushing nose bleed—almost unstoppable. Then I started experiencing them daily for a couple of weeks. Things were now getting complicated, so I began monitoring my blood pressure twice a day; it was elevated just as I had suspected. So between my lower back pain, the unbearable sciatic nerve pain, numbness in my lower limbs, and now uncontrollable nose bleeds and elevated blood pressure, you can see what related health issues can be brought on when living with chronic pain.

This is another reason why it is imperative to do your research as to what to do to reduce and/or eliminate pain.

But no matter my state of mind, I always believed deep inside that I would be healed either supernaturally in a moment by the Great Physician, through natural remedies, or through a human physician.

CHANGES IN ATTITUDE

Living with chronic pain will absolutely affect your attitude. I cannot express just how important it is to maintain or develop a positive attitude or mindset while dealing with a painful condition. We do ourselves more damage by focusing on our pain 24/7 than if we can occupy ourselves with other positive things. Later in the book I address the importance of developing a positive attitude and how negativity can creep in and cause dark thoughts or demonic attacks in a person's mind.

By now, I began feeling more mental stress and developing a negative outlook on finding relief from this pain demon. I have always been a stable, confident, and mentally fit individual, but now, doubt, fear, and uncertainties started to cloud my mind. I could tell my day-to-day thoughts were negatively challenged. This pain demon was getting into my head and affecting my outlook on life. The only pleasurable moments I enjoyed in spite of those painful days was when Lori and I would chill out in our Jacuzzi. In addition to the heated water and jets of bubbles massaging my back muscles, I especially enjoyed the support and understanding I received from Lori. We looked forward to those morning and evening soaks in the tub, and for me it was her presence that made all the difference in overcoming my painful condition.

If you are suffering with chronic pain and you have someone you can trust, who loves you and who will support you when you are down in the dumps, someone who will encourage you with loving kindness and thoughtfulness—count your blessings! Be cautious about focusing too much on yourself and forgetting where others are in all of this. Remember, they are walking with you through your healing process, they too are being affected in many ways, and that was the case with Lori.

MY TRUE HELP METE

Lori, who was so loving and caring day and night, was feeling my pain and hated to see me struggling. As a result, she was wearing down. There were times when she had to get in my face, pointing out that during any conversation regardless of the topic, I would eventually start talking about my pain. It seemed everywhere we went or what we did I was always talking about pain. Many times she would have to tell me to "Stop thinking about pain, all the time...there's more to life... me!" She was right, but my ship was sinking.

Lori and I have always done everything together. We shopped, traveled, worked together; any time you saw Lori, I was somewhere close and vice versa. Little did she know that when we went out for dinner or someone's home I was stressing out inside because going places became a painful experience. The fun in doing even the simplest things in life was beginning to slip away. There was a constant battle of negative and positive thoughts going on in my head. Perhaps I became self-taught when it came to mind over matter because I knew in my heart that I did not want another surgery. I fought the negative attitude daily and kept reminding myself, *The remedy is out there—focus on the purpose not the task.*

PROFESSIONAL STATUS

Besides dealing with attitude issues, I couldn't concentrate on my business. I was losing interest and motivation to keep pushing. Normally I'm the guy who motivates others to stay the course, no matter what. I'm the guy who has positive and encouraging words for others, etc. What was happening to me?

I started canceling TV and radio interviews because I may have slept but a couple hours the night before and looked and felt like a zombie the next early morning. Or just the very thought of walking through another airport to catch another flight and then having to sit for a couple of hours in those uncomfortable, undersized plane seats would cause my hips to inflame. The prospects of being able to face the public with a fresh look on my face and a positive word on my lips was becoming an impossible mountain to scale.

Then the thoughts of not being able to continue my career as a naturopathic doctor, best-selling author, public speaker, and health and fitness professional were crowding out the positive thoughts in my mind. Let's face it, I couldn't convincingly present a seminar about being fit, what foods to eat to stay healthy, how to reach the ideal weight, and the importance of exercise if I didn't look the part. Though I personally live that way, it was also part of the business. I was losing that winner's edge I had always possessed. My mental wellness and fortitude was being attacked and starting to wane to the point that I fought bouts of depression. I was crying inside for help.

I am intentionally being transparent so you know that I know what you may be going through. I want to help you. I have written personal, pertinent material that might help you overcome chronic pain. I want you to have hope and believe you can walk through your healing—and know you are not alone.

Maintaining a healthy lifestyle is crucial. I have kept my body and mind healthy by exercising whether competitively or not, I eat foods based on my blood type, and I take nutritional supplements daily. I spend time in prayer and read the Scriptures daily. I view life as an opportunity to stretch out a canvas and paint the picture of my choice. I believe life has unlimited opportunities for those willing to go after them. I maintain a positive thought process. I love helping others.

It is vitally important for you to develop healthy lifestyle practices and not seek a quick fix. There are no guarantees in life that bad things won't happen to good people; but there's one thing for sure you can depend on, when your body and mind are strong and in balance, there is a greater likelihood for you to rebound when facing an unforeseen injury, disease, or illness.

Sweetheart Cottage

SECTION II

REMEDIES AND SOLUTIONS

CHAPTER 4

THE POWER OF YOUR MIND

"The power of your mind has no limit!" —DR. JOE

In this section I address an area that is least dealt with by most practitioners and medical doctors when it comes to pain management—the significance of the mind, emotions, and attitude. This area, though mostly ignored, is possibly one of the most important aspects of coping with chronic pain and life in general. As is common knowledge in conventional medicine, most doctors are ignorant when it comes to managing pain from the psychological approach and would rather simply write prescriptions for pain medication, a cheaper and less involved approach.

In direct contrast to conventional medicine and its approach to mending chronic pain based on treating symptoms, structural abnormalities, and arthritic degeneration of bone and discs, etc., I examine coping with pain from a more holistic approach, factoring in the whole person. I believe there is place in medicine for both, but here we will explore various techniques, modalities, and methods encompassing the whole person approach for coping with chronic pain.

The importance of positive thinking, the power of your mind to cope with chronic pain, and the role your emotions play are very crucial components to the overall wellness of your life. Each one of these areas of your mind and the role they play in dealing with chronic pain can have a positive or negative effect on your outlook on life, job, relationships, etc. Learning how to apply certain mental exercises for overcoming a painful life is a very crucial component when recovering from surgery, going into surgery, dealing with chronic pain, focusing on your healing process, etc. We all know that words are powerful sounds that roll off our tongues, yet this very small organ, the tongue, can make all the difference in coping with pain or allowing pain to defeat us. This is true because *what you say is what you think.*

So our choice of words is vitally important to the outcome of our goals, desires, and plans. Our words expose what we are really thinking or feeling as well. But how do words affect your level of pain? Could your thoughts actually trigger your pain to flare up?

I'd like to show you how you can cope with pain through the power of your mind, thoughts, and words instead of coping with pain by popping pain meds.

You have probably heard the phrases: "the power of positive persuasion," "think positive and grow rich," and "the power of positive thinking." I agree that there is indeed power in a positive mindset. We need a positive attitude if we plan to reach our goals, finish our education, raise a house full of well-adjusted children, and even overcome pain. But keeping a positive attitude while living with chronic pain is not all that easy, which I will address later in the book.

But right now I want to talk about your brain (not your IQ) and the huge role it plays in pain response. Your brain fulfills this role in two basic ways, through the sensory pathways and the emotional pathways. Most commonly treated by your pain management physician is the Sensory Pathway caused by physical trauma such as an automobile accident, a fall, autoimmune disease, etc. The least treated by pain management and conventional medicine is the Emotional Pathway. This pathway directly affects a person's emotions and responses to both internal and external stimuli (thoughts, words, people, events, etc.) as they play a huge role in inducing painful flare-ups.

With that in mind, I thought it best to first cover this component in coping with chronic pain and then later in this section we can cover the more common natural and alternative remedies, modalities, and treatments for addressing chronic pain. Before we get into all the powerful and beneficial effects you can achieve mentally and emotionally in overcoming a painful condition, I want to share with you a personal experience I had more than once as I was battling with chronic pain. It has to do with the mental dangers associated with the dark side of the mind.

Some people form questionable opinions of those who have been treated for mental health issues. But not all mental issues are a matter of psychosis, neurosis, or being mentally challenged. To reassure you that I feel your pain and the negative thoughts that keep bombarding your mind, I am being very open and transparent about this area and make no apologies for what I experienced. This state of mind makes one very vulnerable. It is very real when overwhelmed and exhausted from chronic pain. I believe the condition of the mind of someone who has been suffering with chronic pain and is exhausted both physically and mentally is open season for demonic attack. This horrifying experience can occur to any individual of sound mind as well, but over time, as chronic pain wears people down, they can slowly forget their purpose and basis for living and start losing all hope for the future. This vulnerable state of the mind can easily come under the influence of demonic attack. And many will succumb to what the voices are saying from the dark side.

NIGHTTIME DEMONIC ATTACKS

Nighttime was worse for me in coping with the pain as well as my emotions. Maybe it was because Lori would be in bed sleeping, and I was up most of the night trying to find a comfortable chair, couch, rug, or any position to give me some relief from the pain demon. Anyone in excruciating chronic pain and sleep-deprived can easily become a vulnerable target for unhealthy thinking. Some may not agree with me making reference to a demonic attack, but when a sound mind is suddenly being darkened by thoughts of committing suicide, there is only one conclusion. This abnormal emotional phenomenon that goes against people's innate and natural fear of pain and death is what happens if they do not guard their minds. But nevertheless, I found myself in battle with these thoughts, thoughts emanating me from the dark side which is undeniably the enemy of my soul, Satan.

I remember one (of many) late nights when I was tossing and turning in pain, so I had to get up. Totally exhausted, I basically crawled toward the couch to lie flat on my back on the floor with my lower legs at a 90-degree angle on the couch to release pressure on my back and hips. I was at my wits' end and thought I was going out of my mind. The pain was so intense; all I could think and focus on was my pain— the mental place where healing and curing cannot exist. That one night in particular, I guess the whole picture of my life was racing through my mind. I just could not take it any longer.

Hundreds of questions were swirling through my mind: *Am I being punished, is this my portion in life, have I been such a terrible person, is Yahweh (God) testing me, punishing me?* I sunk to an all-time low. There I was, Mr. Professional Wellness Guy feeling totally drained, so tired of fighting for and believing that I would find the root cause(s) and remedy to this painful condition and so tired of going through another torturous night without sleep.

There on the floor I broke down in tears and wept. I felt so isolated and alone, so defeated, so discouraged that I wanted to die. While in that mental state I have to say that in all honesty I gave up fending off those thoughts about ending my life. I find it very difficult expressing just what I was feeling as I entertained the thought of committing suicide. I felt like I was almost in a trancelike state of mind. Things were moving slowly. It was very, very eerie. I could feel chills going over my body, my heart racing, and sweat profusely pouring out of my body. *Should I slice my wrists, overdose on the meds, or quickly end it all by shooting my brains out?*

As I mentioned earlier I'm not ashamed to admit this because I know those thoughts were not coming from me; nevertheless, those dark thoughts are very powerful. My mind and body were totally exhausted, the perfect scenario to put me out of my misery. The door of

darkness opened itself for me to walk through. Please be understanding with my transparency and make yourself aware of this possible
horrifying experience, because I know there are others, perhaps you or
someone you know and care about, who may be on that edge also.

As I fought this pain demon I began to pray and ask Yahweh (God)
to please, please heal my body from the pain. I cried out and begged
Him to please take the pain away. Even though He didn't answer my
prayer that night and heal me, He didn't allow the enemy of my soul to
take my life. After the battle in my mind with the dark spirit world had
ended, the next thing I knew it was morning. Yahweh was merciful and
put me to sleep and out of pain for about four or five hours, right there
on the floor. Don't get me wrong, I love my life, I love everything about
it and I have many reasons for living. But living with such level of pain
for so long, I was physically and mentally exhausted and a target for
horrible and destructive thoughts in that condition.

Who said life is fair? It takes the power of your mind plus trust and
reliance on your Creator to see you through your life's journey, at least
it did for me. Let's examine a couple of things that may just be what
you need as you cope with chronic pain.

MIND CONTROL

The concept of "mind over matter" usually appeals to the daredevil
who is ready to lunge off a 250-foot bridge with a bungee cord tied
to his or her ankle, but it can also be appealing to someone who has
totally exhausted every conventional treatment and option to cope with
pain. It is then that the reality of the power of the mind and body connection takes on a hopeful urgency. And I hope it does for you!

Anytime there is a physical injury or trauma that causes pain, the
signal conveying pain travels to the brain via the sensory pathway
and an emotional pathway. This emotional aspect of the experience
of pain travels to (amygdale and the anterior cingulated cortex) your
brain. Mind-body treatments like prayer, meditation, and relaxation
can greatly affect these emotional networks. In fact, researchers have
used functional MRI for chronic pain patients to "visualize" pain.

These images allow a patient to change or manipulate the image and find relief. The individual with chronic pain can become empowered, whether it is through stretching programs, biofeedback, prayer, or meditation. So changing your view of pain can help you better cope with chronic pain.

I have always embraced the power of the mind, or mind over matter. I realize in some circles it may be looked at as somewhat mystical or magical, but the truth is we have been given a mind that is part of our natural makeup; it is powerful and truly capable of overcoming emotional and physical hurdles if we learn to use it.

Some 30 years ago plus, I competed in power lifting competitions. This is where each competitor has to perform three different power lifts: the bench press, the squat (deep knee bend), and the dead lift. Each competitor gets three attempts at each lift, and then the judges tally the heaviest weight lifted per power lift thus establishing the total. Each competitor competed against their totals. I focused on the squat. It seemed to lag behind in ratio to the other two lifts. My primary motive for improving the squat, besides wanting to win the competition, was the fear of getting injured again and pain when squatting. Yes, even we big guys have to deal with fear. Perhaps for me it was due to the time I was crushed with a 650-pound barbell that slid off my shoulders, down my back, and got caught on my support belt buckle that drove me to the floor. I knew if I were ever to improve my squats I would have to change the way I viewed (my thought process) the squat and get over the fear of getting hurt. It would take something more profound than having one of my training partners slap me across my face, which most of them did to each other for an adrenalin rush prior to performing the power lift.

So I taught myself a technique that I call mental imagery or autogenic training. Autogenic training is simply using mental exercises to trigger the relaxation response. It does not use outside stimuli, but is solely a mental exercise. This training produces sensations of warmth and heaviness, which are calming and soothing. It has been successful in treating people who have high blood pressure, migraine headaches, asthma, and sleep disturbances.

It is similar to the mental method of coping with pain through meditation when a person visualizes pain by creating an image that is pleasant or humorous or noisy so it can be turned off (mentally). The idea is to refocus your thought process from the pain onto or into something else, ultimately a distraction. My purpose was to develop a strong mental counterpunch for the fear of injuring myself when placing hundreds of pounds of weight upon my shoulders. I had to view the squat in another way. I envisioned the perfect squat in my mind. This became a vitally important mental exercise I would perform daily besides the grueling workouts in the gym.

To prepare myself for this mental exercise I would actually sit on the floor, rest my back against a wall in a totally comfortable position, close my eyes and take deep slow breaths from my belly, or belly breathing. It took about two minutes or so of deliberate slow breathing for me to relax. At that point I would start concentrating on or visualizing what I thought was the perfect squatting technique. This deep breathing and visualizing technique was something I practiced every day and sometimes twice or more a day. Over time and with much repetition, I could reach that mental imagery visualization of the perfect squat almost on demand.

GETTING RESULTS

The next step was to actually incorporate this mental exercise prior to performing the squat while in the gym training, and eventually in the competition itself. By seeing this perfect squatting technique that I created in my mind, I was becoming less and less fearful of the hundreds of pounds I would have across my shoulders to squat. And an added benefit, by improving my squatting technique, which boosted my confidence, I wasn't second-guessing myself about getting crushed again. I went through my mental routine just before my name was called to go out on the lifting platform to perform the squat. The end result was twofold. My newly improved squatting technique plus newfound confidence caused me to achieve a personal best for weight in the squat; and perhaps most importantly, I overcame fear, my primary mental enemy. This is the same approach I have used when dealing with pain, particularly when it was spiking.

As I explored all the many treatments and modalities for ridding my body of chronic pain, I believe it was the mental side of physical pain that helped me reduce and sometimes squelch it. In fact, this allowed me to deal with pain much better and at the same time helped me stay more mentally calm and at ease. When taking various medications we are actually just treating the symptoms and never discovering the root cause of the pain. For some people, they experience a placebo effect from taking medications, and they feel better. A placebo effect is very powerful and convincing, but it does not remove the pain—your mind does, which is supporting evidence that the mind is capable of helping us overcome almost anything life brings our way.

Depending on dangerous, health-damaging pain medications for long periods of time is counterproductive to coping with pain mentally, with your mind. When your mind is trained to take away the pain or cause a mental disturbance from the pain, it becomes an obvious coping tool for chronic pain. And to boot, using your mind doesn't cost you a single penny or loss of health. Surely you want to use the power of your mind and avoid all the potential health-related problems, and potential premature death, from pain medications.

It is important to understand that negative emotions such as anxiety, stress, and anger can cause flare-ups or spikes in your pain level; yet if you take control of your mind and thoughts, you can actually reduce the pain level, or put the fire out so to speak. You must remember that you are capable of overcoming pain, fear, or anything else if you put your mind to it.

Coping with your pain is as mental as it is physical—and maybe more. Some say that chronic pain is 80 percent mental (emotional pathway) and 20 percent physical (sensory pathway). Now isn't that a twist in what you've been told all these painful years. To imagine the majority of our pain, real physical pain is more mental than physical is hard to believe. That is because we all have been taught to listen to conventional teaching and modalities and treatments from conventional medicine. Just imagine if you started practicing some mental exercises, which you could do at home anytime day or night. Just imagine how successful you would be in all aspects of your life. This is the difference between conventional medicine thinking and holistic medicine thinking, which considers the "whole person."

In holistic medicine (vs. conventional medicine) the patient participates in the healing process, which brings together the body-mind connection. In conventional medicine all the patient has to do is visit the doctor, get a prescription for pain, and pop the pills. But what approach do you use when you are experiencing various emotions like nervousness, fear, anger, or anxiety? We know that negative emotions can induce your pain level, increase your nervousness, and eventually put you in a state of anxiety and perhaps a panic attack. When pain spikes or flares up physically, immediately your mind comes into play. You start imagining the worst. You start focusing on the pain, which disrupts any hope of healing or calming. When you have a flare-up, you begin to think negative or worrisome thoughts like, *How am I am going to make it to the party tonight,* or *I'm going to have another setback,* or *I'm going to end up needing a walker for the rest of my life,* or *I feel another panic attack coming on.* I'm sure if you have chronic pain, you have experienced those flare-up incidents and negative thoughts on a regular basis. And if you are like most people who are dealing with chronic pain, you will probably reach for some pain pills to reduce the pain.

It's time to change your thinking, now!

I can attest to the fact that there were many occasions when I had some pressing event or appointments or simply had guests or even family members come over to our house and I would experience a flare-up in pain. It was like my mind would go into an inflammation mode. And the irony of it all—if I took a pain med for the inflammation, it did no good. I would get aggravated because I got no relief from the pain meds, and the pain got worse. What a constant mental ping-pong game of trying to cope with chronic pain. But the interesting thing was, as I started applying some of the mental exercises I am about you share with you, I was able to better handle the pain plus enjoy life even though I was still dealing with chronic pain. The difference was, *instead of the pain controlling my mind, I taught my mind to control the pain!* When I changed or refocused my thoughts from the pain itself, I was able to cause it to subside to a very manageable level or even eliminate it completely.

Here's a simple mind-body technique protocol that you might want to perfect. It will work; but be patient as you are retraining your thinking and learning anew.

MIND CHANGE—PAIN CHANGE

To start, get into a comfortable sitting or lying position. I know when you are in pain that is sometimes impossible, so get creative. Use a pillow or a pad under your knees if you are lying down or use your favorite chair, the couch, or whatever you need to get into a comfortable position.

If possible perform this exercise alone so there are no distractions. Any such coping technique for chronic pain should begin with controlled deep breathing:

1. Wear loose clothing so you can breathe without restriction.

2. Settle into a relaxed position in a dark room.

3. Close your eyes or focus on a central point.

4. Breathe in deeply and exhale slowly while continuing to focus.

5. Continue with deep, slow breathing for a few minutes.

6. Don't force this technique. It will take practice to perfect it but you can.

Examples of mental imagery/chronic pain control techniques:

1. Focus on a project, goal, or the greatest vacation imaginable; the idea is to divert the mind away from focusing on the pain.

2. Create a mental image of an ice pack that numbs the painful body part; focus on numbing and how that takes away the pain.

3. Create a mental image of pain as being a fire. Watch yourself put the fire out with a fire hose.

4. Think what it was like when you were pain-free, focus on being pain-free.

5. Focus on something or someone who makes you laugh.

6. Silently, count *all* your blessings, which helps divert pain from the mind.

I know these examples may sound weird, but they work. Take your time and soon you will be able to create mental imagery. You will be training your mind to divert or distract itself whenever you have a flare-up or feel pain. I have been able to divert my thoughts from pain many times by mental imagery. I suggest that you work on mental imagery starting at five minutes and eventually reaching 30 minutes three times per week.

I have several different mental/emotional techniques or diversions when coping with chronic pain. I love comedy, and for me the old reruns of *Seinfeld* and the *King of Queens* keep me laughing. On the more serious side is emotional healing that comes from daily prayer and counting my blessings. I will also sing and whistle around the house when I am trying to divert my attention from pain. It seems the more often I divert my mind from pain, the better I keep pain manageable. Developing your own means of diversion will also help you avoid popping another pain pill that is only treating the symptom.

RECAP

Remember to relax yourself, practice slow, deliberate, deep inhaling and exhaling. When focusing on pain, immediately *stop!* Switch your mind to one of your diversions. Divert all negativity by mental imagery of pleasant or humorous diversions. Get rid of the old way of coping with pain by practice, practice, and more practice.

CHAPTER 5

Deep Breathing to Control Pain

"You could be just a breath away from pain—free living!" —Dr. Joe

Everything about the human body is interrelated, so I want to explain further about the importance of deep breathing. I believe you will find it very interesting and also very useful as you are walking through your healing. I touched on how to prepare for mental imagery by practicing deep breathing so to relax your body, nervous system, and mind so you can create a mental diversion from your pain. But now we'll go much further and see how slow, deep breathing affects your health, attitude, and pain.

Did you know you can live seven days without water? Did you know you can live more than 50 days without food? Did you know you can't live more than five minutes or so without oxygen? Those facts alone tell us how important it is to better understand how essential breathing is for our survival and overall good health. That is why I would tell my clients during exercise class not to hold their breath, as some had a tendency to do. It is important to breathe!

It is interesting to know that when our immune system becomes overactive we can be susceptible to breathing disorders such as asthma, emphysema, and interstitial lung diseases. But when proper breathing is practiced on a regular basis, not only does the immune system benefit but the brain does as well. Japanese studies show us that during relaxed abdominal breathing, brain waves also show a pattern of relaxation. In addition, heart rate variability (HRV) has been studied extensively. Poor HRV has been linked with increased mortality after a heart attack. It's very interesting that poor heart rate variability has also been linked to depression, anger, and anxiety—the very emotions that can trigger pain, cause pain to flare up, and disrupt the healing process. Research has found that proper breathing can improve HRV and reduce immune activation.

In conclusion, a concerted effort in focusing on our breathing can produce a rhythmic pattern of healthy heart rate variability and a healthy immune function result. And that means a longer and healthier life.[1]

USING BREATHING TO REDUCE PAIN

For cancer patients, you can learn to use breathing exercises to shift your focus away from pain.[2] The human mind processes one thing at a time. If you focus on the rhythm of your breathing, you're not focused on the pain. The moment we anticipate pain, most of us tend to stop breathing and hold our breath. Holding our breath activates the fight/flight/freeze response and it tends to increase the sensation of pain, stiffness, anxiety, or fear. So instead of holding your breath when fearful or anticipating pain, exhale instead.

THE VAGUS NERVE

Your body's levels of stress hormones are regulated by the *autonomic nervous system* (ANS).[3] The ANS has two components that balance each other, the sympathetic nervous system (SNS) and the parasympathetic nervous system (PNS). The SNS turns up your nervous system. It helps us handle the flight-or-fight response; whereas the PNS turns down the nervous system to help calm us and enhances relaxation, rest, sleep, and drowsiness by slowing our heart rate and breathing. This is where you want to teach your body to take you for better coping with pain and healing.

The *vagus nerve* is the nerve that comes from the brain and controls the parasympathetic nervous system that controls your relaxation response. This nervous system uses the neurotransmitter, acetylcholine. If your brain cannot communicate with your diaphragm via the release of acetylcholine from the vagus nerve (for example, impaired by botulinum toxin), then you will stop breathing and die.[4]

Acetylcholine is responsible for learning and memory. It is also calming and relaxing, which is used by the vagus nerve to send messages of peace and relaxation throughout your body. New research has found that acetylcholine is a major brake on inflammation in the body.[5] In other words, stimulating your vagus nerve sends acetylcholine throughout your body, not only relaxing you but also turning down the fires of inflammation that are related to the negative effects from stress.[6]

Because I have had very good results with adult adipose stem cells for my back, neck, and hips problems, it's exciting to see that new research has also linked the vagus nerve to improved neurogenesis, increased BDNF output (brain-derived neurotropic factor is like super fertilizer for your brain cells) and repair of brain tissue, and to actual regeneration throughout the body. For example, scientists[7] have found that stems cells are directly connected to the vagus nerve. Activating the vagus nerve can stimulate stem cells to produce new cells and repair and rebuild your own organs.

There are many ways to activate the vagus nerve and turn on the relaxation response. When you take a deep breath and relax and expand your diaphragm, your vagus system is stimulated, you instantly turn on the parasympathetic nervous system, your cortisol levels are reduced, pain levels drop, and your brain heals.

THREE TYPES OF BREATHING

As Dr. Mark Liponis[8] describes, there are three types of breathing:

Clavicular breathing—A breath that comes from high up in the shoulders and collarbones

Chest breathing—A breath that comes from the center of the chest

Abdominal breathing—A breath that comes from the abdomen

The first breathing pattern uses the collarbone (the clavicle) to help move air. You see it most often in people who are feeling panicked, or who truly are struggling for breath, as those with emphysema often do. Clavicular breathing is the most abnormal form of breathing. It occurs with serious breathing impairment or during extreme stress—such as during a panic attack.

The second breathing pattern is the most common. Your chest and lungs will be expanding, but the expansion is restricted by tension and tightness in the muscles around the abdomen and ribs. This causes the chest to expand mainly upward, with less airflow and more rapid respiration.

The third kind of breath comes from the abdomen and uses the diaphragm. When the diaphragm contracts, your lungs expand, pulling air in through your mouth like bellows. When you breathe from your abdomen, your belly will expand and move out with each inhalation. Your chest will rise slightly, but not nearly as much as with chest breathing; your abdomen is doing all the moving.

Through abdominal breathing you can activate vagus nerve and trigger a *relaxation response*. The relaxation response, which is the opposite of the *stress response*, is necessary for your body to heal, repair, and renew.

HOW TO ACTIVATE THE VAGUS NERVE YOURSELF

To practice deep breathing, inhale through your nose and exhale through your mouth. Remember to:

- Breathe more slowly.

- Breathe more deeply, from the belly.

- Exhale longer than you inhale.[9]

You can proceed as follows: take a breath into your belly (expanding your diaphragm) to the count of five or so, pause for a second then breathe out slowly by keeping your lips tight. While at rest most people take about 10 to 14 breaths per minute.[10] Ideally, reduce your breathing to 5 to 7 times per minute. Exhaling through your mouth instead of the nose makes your breathing a conscious process, not a subconscious one.

As you do this, your muscles will relax, dropping your worries and anxieties. The oxygen supply to your body's cells increases and this helps produce endorphins, the body's feel-good hormones. Deep breathing reduces the effects of stress, helps fight depression, lowers blood pressure, heart rate and boosts the immune systems.

CHAPTER 6

TMS:
TENSION MYOSITIS SYNDROME

"When I complained of an ache or pain as a kid, my mother would say, "Its all in your head!" —DR. JOE

Let's explore another vehicle for addressing chronic pain. Just as we looked into the power of the mind and by performing simple but viable mental exercises, you will develop the mental power to control chronic pain, a healthier non-medicated means for coping. With a different approach, let's see what may be causing the chronic pain you are experiencing. Perhaps the root cause may be all in your head.

Think about this for a moment, have you ever been insulted, criticized, or even felt unappreciated and allowed your hurt feelings to fester in your mind? You have never confronted those feelings by speaking to the person who inflicted them; you hid them deep down inside. Or perhaps you have been holding ill feelings toward an incapacitated loved one for whom you were a caretaker for many years. Perhaps deep inside you resent the person for taking all your time. There are many scenarios that may come to your mind—and these feelings are quite normal; they are, in fact, universal.

We "repress our feelings" for a variety of reasons and many may be hidden way down inside in our vault—the unconscious mind. Unintentionally we taught ourselves to harbor various emotional feelings

67

and consequently our unconscious mind has been at war with our conscious mind to expel the repressed emotions until, over time, we begin to experience certain manifestations like illness, disease, and even chronic pain.

In naturopathy we consider our brain to be similar to an electrical power plant. From the brain travel electrical currents and impulses that go into our liver that manufactures DNA and many other components for balancing a healthy life. We know that when there is a break in the electrical circuit from the brain to the liver, our health will be impaired and possible complications will occur if left unaddressed. Unresolved emotions, one of the main "circuit breakers," are responsible for premature health problems via illness, disease, and chronic pain.

In other words, if you been hurt by someone and believe you have gotten over the hurt, yet when the person's name comes up in conversation you get red in the face and all kind of negative emotions start swirling around in your head, then, my friend, that is a sign you have repressed painful emotions. As we keep them repressed, they can show up as chronic pain.

In his book, *Healing Back Pain, the Mind/Body Connection*, Dr. John E. Sarno, MD, explains Tension Myositis Syndrome (TMS) for treating his patients for chronic pain in the neck, shoulder, back, and buttock.[1] Conventional medical training taught him that these types of conditions were probably due to abnormalities of the spine, arthritis, and disc disorders or a group of muscle conditions attributed to poor posture, under-exercise, overexertion, etc. Conventional treatments are injections, deep heat in the form of ultrasound, massage, and exercise. This was frustrating to Dr. Sarno because the pattern of pain and examination findings didn't always correlate to the reason for pain. For instance, a patient may have pain in places that had nothing to do with bones when they showed degenerative arthritic changes in the lower end of their spine on a magnetic resonance imaging (MRI).

Something else that caused him to perfect TMS treatments was his findings that about 88 percent of people with these issues also had histories of tension or migraine headaches, heartburn, hiatus hernia, stomach ulcer, colitis, spastic colon, irritable bowel syndrome (IBS), hay fever, asthma, eczema, etc., all related to tension. He believed their condition might also be induced by tension. This is the basis of Tension Myositis Syndrome (*myo* means muscle and *sitis* means inflammation). TMS is defined as a change of state in the muscle that is painful.[2]

The primary muscle groups by which TMS are commonly found are the larger muscles; buttocks muscle (gluteal), low back (lumbar muscles), and upper shoulders (trapezius muscles). Secondary muscles are the neck and top of the shoulders. With the hypothesis being that the pain syndrome originates in the brain rather than in some abnormality in spine or incompetence of muscles, it only makes sense that regardless of an MRI or X-ray reading showing a herniated disc or stenosis of the back, or spinal degeneration, etc., doesn't necessarily mean that those areas are the pain generators.

Because TMS is least pursued by conventional medicine, you may have never heard of it or can vaguely see its correlation with repressed emotions and how those repressed emotions manifest themselves in areas of the body that express true physical pain. After a thorough examination of the patient to rule out structural, organic, or genetic causes for pain, the patient is then tested for having TMS. Once the patient tests positive for TMS, a series of consultations and classroom participation is scheduled. The patients are taught the correlation between chronic pain and repressed emotions, such as anger and anxiety, and how it manifests in the larger muscles of the body as well as ligaments and tendons.

I know it may sound weird to imagine that repressed emotions can be the cause of your painful lower back, but they can be! Many people reject the notion of this disorder until they find themselves desperate after trying everything else. Understanding that our unconscious mind is always working toward unloading those painful emotional experiences, yet the other side of our brain, the conscious mind, is not allowing those painful emotions to be dealt with creates a constant conflict within us. Then there is the added uncomfortableness of thinking we have some emotional disorder that our society frowns upon regarding mental health issues.

I personally find Dr. Sarno's approach to healing chronic pain for those who have TMS very enlightening and also may be the very solution to your chronic pain. I strongly suggest if you have tried everything else for chronic pain and have flare-ups that cripple you with pain that may be connected with something emotional like stressful circumstances, a traumatic incident, or hurt feelings, it may be wise to read his book. Perhaps you will discover one more clue to destroying the pain demon you have been struggling with for way too long.

As you walk through your healing, keep in mind that even if you haven't found that particular treatment or remedy to remove the pain or reached your full healing yet, there is a light at the end of the tunnel. Let's keep walking together and see what things you can be doing to avoid the onset of certain conditions from a preventative perspective, as well as what to do to enhance your recovery to normal healthy living.

SECTION III

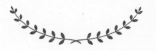

IDENTIFICATION

CHAPTER 7

MAP YOUR CHOICES

"Maps are good for preventing wrong turns!" —DR. JOE

One of my major concerns for people with musculoskeletal pain, chronic pain, or even pain from auto accidents, falls, degenerative diseases, physical traumas, etc., is being aware of what treatments and protocols in conventional medicine and alternative medicine are available and which ones would best suit their needs. Of course my first and foremost suggestion is to try every treatment possible to avoid surgery.

Musculoskeletal conditions, or disorders, affect the body's muscles, joints, tendons, ligaments, bones, and nerves. The pain and discomfort associated with these conditions can create limited physical functioning that can affect the overall quality of life.

The first step in mapping your choices is to carefully read Chart A and Chart B within this chapter. Then read Section IV, Treatment Options, in its entirety, including the Glossary of Treatments. By reviewing this material, the charts and glossary, you will have better insights to the treatments and procedures for your particular condition. Once you feel you have made the accurate decision, contact a reliable healthcare practitioner or physician to assist you in receiving maximum results.

In the 8 Simple Steps to a Pain-Free and Healthy Life section, you will learn many different healthy lifestyle practices to help you strengthen your immune system and overall health. I believe when our body is physically fit, it is more resilient and can bounce back after an injury to a joint or when illness strikes. If your physician suggests rehabilitation after surgery, a healthier body will make it much easier to recover. A healthier body, stronger immune system, and better conditioned muscles serve as preventative measures to offset painful musculoskeletal conditions. Having a healthier body may lessen the pain from:

- Knee and Achilles tendon injuries

- Tendon tears

- Trauma injuries such as sprains, joint dislocations, and fractures

- Back and neck

- Sore shoulders

- Pinched nerves

- Osteoporosis

- Arthritis

- Bone tumors

- Repetitive stress injuries such as tendonitis and carpal tunnel syndrome

- Joint injury

COMMON TREATMENTS FOR MUSCULOSKELETAL DISORDERS

An individual can experience decreased pain while regaining optimal strength, mobility, and overall physical functioning with various treatments. Here are just a few common treatments:

- Physical and occupational therapy

- Injections with anti-inflammatory drugs and/or pain medications

- Therapeutic massage and osteopathic manipulation

- Patient-centered care

Certainly this list is very limited, but as mentioned very common. My goal is to make available to you modalities or treatment options other than what is mainstream. In other words, when you are diagnosed with a certain musculoskeletal problem or condition, your condition may require 1) a surgical procedure, 2) a medical non-surgical procedure, or 3) a natural, alternative, non-surgical procedure for relief of pain. Your choice will have a direct impact on the quality of life that follows, so being certain of your decision makes good sense. In our Western societal and cultural mindset, most people automatically choose conventional medicine and surgery as a first line of defense— unaware of the many natural alternatives available, which may be the very modality they need.

AMERICA SPEAKS: PAIN IN AMERICA

A nationwide survey[1] assessed Americans view of pain, gauging their perceptions of how pain sufferers and the medical community deal with chronic pain. The following is from the survey:

> Among the major adjustments that chronic pain sufferers have made are such serious steps as taking disability leave from work (20%), changing jobs altogether (17%), getting help with activities of daily living (13%), and moving to a home that is easier to manage (13%).

A Visit to the Doctor

- Most pain sufferers (63%) have seen their family doctor for help.

- 40 percent made an appointment with a specialist, such as an orthopedist.

- 25 percent have visited a chiropractor or a doctor that specializes in pain management (15%).

- While 43% of pain sufferers have been to only one type of doctor for their pain, a large proportion (38%) have

consulted more than one practitioner in the medical
community.

- Treatments for pain have yielded mixed results.
Although 58% of those who took prescription medication
say that doing so was fairly effective for their pain, only
41% of those who took over-the-counter medication experienced the same relief.

The Pain Gap

Seven in ten Americans feel that pain research and management should be one of the medical community's top few
priorities (16%) or a high priority (55%).

Almost six in 10 adults (57%) say they would be willing to pay
one dollar more per week in taxes to increase federal funding
for the scientific research into the causes and treatment of pain.

PAIN GENERATORS

As you are dealing with chronic pain or acute pain, sometimes the
location of the pain can be tricky. In other words, you may have a very
painful joint, but the pain may not be coming from that particular joint,
even though that is where it hurts.

Most patients assume that the doctor knows best; therefore they are
vulnerable to his or her "opinion" and become victims of the wrong
diagnosis and prognosis. Let's face it, if you needed a lawyer, you certainly want one who has won lots of cases! Well the same applies when
selecting a doctor, especially a surgeon. Without placing blame but for
simplicity purposes only, let's assume your doctor is an orthopedic surgeon who examined the hip joint(s) and recommended an MRI. Upon
the radiologist's report, your doctor made a prognosis and suggests hip
replacement surgery. But most people do not realize that MRI photos
do not tell the whole story; and unfortunately the patient may take the
doctor's advice and have hip replacement surgery. Had the patient been
better informed, he or she would know that there may be other sources

of pain or "pain generators" as the underlying painful hip joint. This knowledge could very well have saved the patient from having unnecessary hip replacement surgery.

When you are willing to test everything else first, request other examinations as well as specialists for additional opinions pertaining to conditions such as spinal nerve impingement, bulging discs, muscle spasms, and examination of the surrounding soft tissue or connective tissue of the joint(s), the ligaments and tendons that hold the joints in place to function normally. Because ligaments connect bone to bone and support the integrity of the joint function and movement, and tendons connect muscle to bone and are the musculature that helps support the joint also, it is imperative to thoroughly examine all potential pain generators for the root cause of the pain.

Even though the patient may experience excruciating pain in a particular joint, the problem may not be that joint. The pain could be what is commonly called referred pain. Referred pain comes from a pain generator in another area in the body but creates a painful sensation in a specific joint. For example, if a person injured his pelvic ligaments or tendons which didn't heal properly or if a woman after pregnancy starts having sacroiliac joint (SI) joint or hip pain, the actual pain generator may very well be the pelvis ligaments or tendons that were overstretched or did not heal properly. Consequently the overstretched tendon or ligament became lax and weak. In this case, the hip joints lose their integrity and become unstable or sloppy. This unstable joint (this applies to any joint) would be very painful when the patient stood up or performed normal joint movements like walking, bending, or extending—yet the hip joint is not the problem. The problem is in the ligaments or tendons. How horrible to have had a hip replaced when there was no need—and you still have the same pain!

By palpating or creating pressure on the ligaments and tendons there is an immediate sensation of pain as that is an area or hot spot where the tissue has been damaged or improperly healed. So to help relieve the pain in the hips, the connective tissue requires several treatments to rejuvenate and repair the fibrous tissue. The most effective procedure for accomplishing this condition is referred to as Regenerative Orthopedics (Prolotherapy). Once the ligaments and tendons heal properly and became tight, they in turn support the integrity and function of the hip joint, and the hip pain soon diminishes or disappears. This, in conjunction with a rehabilitation program, can do wonders for your road to recovery and greater quality of life.

So if you are contemplating surgery for your hips (or any joint), please test everything else first! Make the time to exhaust all other treatments before having surgery.

Recap: when you have exhausted all natural and alternative treatments and still experience severe pain and disability, surgery may be your only choice. Be very selective in the surgeon you choose. Take time to get several options and any referrals from patients of the surgeon you are contemplating. It will bring comfort to know your surgeon who "specializes and is very experienced" in their craft, has a good batting average!

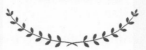

MUSCULOSKELETAL CONDITIONS SYMPTOMS, ROOT CAUSES AND PROCEDURES

RHEUMATOID ARTHRITIS (RA)

Rheumatoid arthritis (RA) is an autoimmune disease where the body's immune system attacks its own joints and joint tissue. RA can cause inflammation of the joints and joint tissues. RA is characterized by flare-ups and remissions and can affect multiple joints or singular joints. When inflammation is chronic, the disease can cause joint destruction and deformity.

Symptoms

The symptoms are painful swelling of the joints, stiffness, and joint dysfunction. Joint damage or degeneration can occur from RA.

Root Cause

RA occurs from an overactive immune system response.

Treatment Options

Natural—Non-Surgical Procedures

- Stem cell/PRP (platelet rich plasma) injections
- Regenerative Orthopedics (Prolotherapy) injections
- Chinese herbal medicine and herbal patches

- Food selections based on blood type
- Apitherapy (bee venom therapy)
- Exercise—stretching, water exercises/aerobics
- Nutritional supplementation

Medical—Non-Surgical Procedures

- Medications

OSTEOARTHRITIS

Osteoarthritis describes the changes that occur in joints as we age. Osteoarthritis is referred to as arthritis of the hips (spine), wear and tear arthritis, or degenerative joint disease. Over time, in the joints of hips or knees, which are weight-bearing joints, there is the wearing away of the cartilage, the protective material between bone on bone. Over time, some of the changes can be in the form of narrowing of the spinal joints, cysts, and bone spurs. Osteoarthritis causes aches and stiffness in the lower back.

Symptoms
Stiffness, pain, or aches in the lower back

Root Causes
Fractures from traumas and aging

Treatment Options
Natural—Non-Surgical Procedures

- Stem cell/PRP (platelet rich plasma) injections
- Regenerative Orthopedics (Prolotherapy) injections
- Chinese herbal medicine and herbal patches
- Food selections based on blood type
- Physical Therapy (PT)
- Dietary supplementation
- Acupuncture

- Apitherapy (bee venom therapy)
- Chiropractic care

Medical—Non-Surgical Procedures

- Medications

OSTEOPOROSIS OF THE SPINE

Osteoporosis of the spine is a painful degenerative condition that is a result of bone loss density. This condition causes weakened bones, making them very susceptible to fractures from falls. Osteoporosis is common among the elderly and women, and occurs in the hips and spine.

Symptoms

- Curvature of the spine; loss of normal height
- Pain brought on by fractured bone

Root Causes

- Menopause
- Aging process
- Falls or trauma
- Lack of calcium, Vitamin D
- Imbalance in pH, acidosis
- Imbalance of hormones

Treatment Options

Natural—Non-Surgical Procedures

- Stem cell/PRP (platelet rich plasma) injections
- Regenerative Orthopedics (Prolotherapy) injections
- Food selection based on blood type; balance pH
- Chinese herbal medicine and herbal patches
- Hormonal Replacement Treatment (HRT), nutritional supplements

- Acupuncture

Medical—Non-Surgical Procedures

- Medications

STENOSIS (BACK)

Stenosis is a narrowing of the spinal canal or the Foramen. This area or opening allows the nerve roots to pass through unrestricted. When degeneration occurs like cysts, bone spurs, and even collapsed discs, the opening starts narrowing and causes pain and pressure on the nerve roots, or the spinal cord. This narrowing can occur anywhere in the spinal column.

Symptoms

- **Cervical Spine (neck)**: Tightness in the neck; pain traveling down the arms into the fingers and hands; difficulty using hands; loss of strength due to pain, numbness.
- **Lumbar Spine**: Lower body, buttocks, and legs feel heavy or weak. Walking for long periods causes pain. Numbness and weakness and cramping in the lower limbs are associated stenosis in the lumbar spine.

Root Causes

- **Cervical Spine (neck)**: Degenerative changes such as bone spurs or arthritic buildup that press against nerves. Herniated discs can cause pressure or compression on the nerves.
- **Lumbar Spine**: Less spinal canal space for nerves to pass freely; narcosis or lack of blood flow.

Treatment Options

Natural—Non-Surgical Procedures

- Physical therapy, anti-gravity stretches

- Stem cell/PRP (platelet rich plasma) injections
- Regenerative Orthopedics (Prolotherapy) injections
- Chinese herbal medicine and herbal patches
- Food selection based on blood type
- Acupuncture

Medical—Non-Surgical Procedures

- Spinal Epidural, Cortisone injections
- Pain and/or anti-inflammatory medications

Medical—Surgical Procedures (only when all else fails)

- **Cervical Laminectomy**: Removal of lamina and spinous process to relieve pressure, pain on spinal cord (neck)
- **Surgical Decompression**: Easing the pressure on the nerve roots or spinal cord by removing bone spurs and/or portions of the lamina or enlarging the foramina
- **Posterolateral Fusion**: Stabilizing the spine with screws and rods
- **Anterior Lumbar Interbody Fusion (ALIF)**: Surgically replacing the damaged disc with a spacer with bone graft. An advanced decompression surgery through the abdomen.
- **Posterior Transformal Interbody Fusion:** Same as ALIF except approach is through the back. Pedicle screws are used to assist in fusion of the vertebral joints.

DEGENERATIVE DISC DISEASE

Degenerative Disc Disease (DDD) is referred to as arthritis of the back and occurs in many people during the normal aging process. As a person ages, these shock-absorbing pads or discs found between the vertebral bodies tend to collapse upon one another due to loss of elasticity. The nerve roots, or spinal cord, are compressed, causing local and radiating pain from the back down one or both legs.

Symptoms

- Radiating pain traveling into legs and feet
- Pain worsens with long periods of standing or sitting
- Throbbing pain in lower back
- Stiffness in lower back

Root Causes

- Obesity; additional pressure on the joints, discs, nerves
- Heavy, repetitive lifting; improper lifting
- Injury, trauma
- Change in formation of disc, normal aging process
- Smoking

Treatment Options

Natural—Non-Surgical Procedures

- Physical therapy, anti-gravity stretches
- Core exercises; enhances stability and support
- Stem Cell/PRP (platelet rich plasma) injections
- Regenerative Orthopedics (Prolotherapy) injections
- Chinese herbal medicine and herbal patches
- Food selections based on blood type
- Acupuncture
- Chiropractic care

Medical—Non-Surgical Procedures

- Spinal Epidural, Cortisone injections

- Medications

Medical—Surgical Procedures (only when all else fails)

- **Surgical Decompression**: Easing the pressure on the nerve roots or spinal cord by removing bone spurs and/or portions of the lamina or enlarging the foramina.

- **Disc Replacement**: Removal of dysfunctional disc with artificial prosthesis.

- **Posterolateral Fusion**: Stabilizing the spine with screws and rods.

- **Anterior Lumbar Interbody Fusion (ALIF)**: Surgically replacing the damaged disc with a spacer with bone graft. An advanced decompression surgery through the abdomen.

- **Posterior Transformal Interbody Fusion**: Same as ALIF except the approach is through the back. Pedicle screws are used to assist in fusion of the vertebral joints.

SPONDYLOLISTHESIS

The slippage of one vertebral body upon another due to arthritis, fracture, trauma is referred to as spondylolisthesis. This condition can cause nerve symptoms due to slippage and spinal instability.

Symptoms

- Pain in lower back
- Referred or leg pain
- Numbness in leg(s)

Root Cause

Usually inherited at childhood or adolescence

Treatment Options

Natural—Non-Surgical Procedures

- Physical therapy, core exercises
- Stem Cell/PRP (platelet rich plasma) injections
- Regenerative Orthopedics (Prolotherapy) injections
- Chinese herbal medicine and herbal patches
- Food selections based on blood type

Medical—Non-Surgical Procedures

- Pain medications
- Spinal Epidural, Cortisone injections

Medical—Surgical Procedures (only when all else fails)

SCIATICA

Sciatica is nerve pain that travels from the spine down one or both legs below the knee(s) and into the feet. Sciatica causes numbness, tingling, and even weakness in the legs. It is referred to as either inflammation or compression of one or more of the branches of the sciatica nerve.

Symptoms

Searing or burning sensation

Root Causes

- Compression of piriformis or gluteus muscles of the buttocks impinging on the branch nerve
- Occurs in the lower back (spine/discs) and/or sacrum deep into the gluteus muscles
- Impingement of bulging discs or narrowing of nerve canal/stenosis
- The sciatica nerve can be inflamed from continual impingement or pressure.

Treatment Options

Natural—Non-Surgical Procedures

- Physical therapy, core exercises, stretching
- Stem Cell/PRP (platelet rich plasma) injections
- Regenerative Orthopedics (Prolotherapy) injections
- Chinese herbal medicine and herbal patches
- Food selections based on blood type
- Acupuncture
- Chiropractic care

Medical—Non-Surgical Procedures

- Pain medications
- Spinal Epidural, Cortisone injections

Medical—Surgical Procedures (only when all else fails)

HERNIATED DISC

The rupture of a piece of a disc is referred to as a herniated disc. A herniated disc is sometimes referred to as a bulging or degenerative disc and causes pressure on the spinal cord or nerves.

Symptoms

Radiating or traveling pain down one or both legs and/or arms causing numbness and/or weakness.

Root Causes

- Collapsed disc
- Weak vertebral ligaments
- Poor posture, improper heavy lifting
- Accident or trauma

Treatment Options

Natural—Non-Surgical Procedures

- Physical therapy
- Stem Cell/PRP (platelet-rich plasma) injections
- Regenerative Orthopedics (Prolotherapy) injections
- Chinese herbal medicine and herbal patches
- Food selections based on blood type
- Acupuncture
- Chiropractic care

Medical—Non-Surgical Procedures

- Pain medications
- Spinal Epidural, Cortisone injections

Medical—Surgical Procedures (only when all else fails)

TUMORS

All tumors are either malignant or benign. Attached to the spinal vertebrae they are part of secondary deposition of malignant or benign tumors from other organs.

Symptoms
None

Root Causes
Adhesions from other organs

Treatments

Natural—Non-Surgical Procedures

- Personal Illness Profiling (PIP); herbal remedies
- Food selections based on blood type

Medical—Surgical Procedures (only when all else fails)

- Radiation

- Chemotherapy

INFECTIONS

Infections occur when discs and spinal bones pick up bacteria from urine or blood.

Symptoms

- Achy pain
- Fever, tenderness

Root Causes

Bacteria from urine or blood

Treatment Options

Natural—Non-Surgical Procedures

- Personal illness profiling (PIP); herbal remedies
- Chinese herbal medicine and herbal patches
- Food selection based on blood type

Medical—Surgical Procedures (only when all else fails)

- Antibiotics
- Possible surgery

CHART B

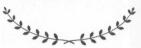

INJURIES

HIPS

Hip pain is a common problem and can be confusing as there are several causes. It is important to have an accurate diagnosis of the cause of your symptoms (not just the symptoms) so the appropriate modality or treatment can be directed at the root cause. The hip joints are more complicated than other joints and therefore should have a thorough examination including the soft tissue or connective tissue that supports the joint—before determining what treatment is necessary.

Symptoms

- Sharp pain
- Burning pain
- Pain on the outside of the hip joint (greater trochanter)
- Pain on the inside of the hip joint (groin)
- Difficulty walking, aggravated by prolonged sitting and standing

Root Causes

- **Arthritis**: The most common and frequent cause of hip pain. There are many natural treatments available. If all else fails, then hip replacement may be your only option.

- **Trochanteric Bursitis**: A very common condition that causes inflammation of the bursa over the outside of the hip joint.

- **Tendonitis**: Can happen in any of the tendons that attach to the hip joint. The most common area where tendonitis occurs is around the hip, where the iliotibial band (IT band) attaches. It is commonly referred to as iliotibial band tendonitis.

- **Osteonecrosis**: A condition that occurs when the blood flow to an area of a bone is disrupted or restricted. Without sufficient blood flow, the cells die off and the bone can collapse. This is common with someone with hip pain.

- **Referred Pain, Lumbar Pain**: Pain that is felt in the buttocks and hips many times can come from the spinal cord. This usually means a disc is herniated and/or sciatica nerve impingement.

- **Snapping Hip Syndrome**: This condition causes a loud snapping sound and can occur in three areas: 1) where the IT band snaps over the outside of the thigh, 2) where torn cartilage of the hip socket and/or labrum tears cause a snapping feeling, and 3) hip flexor snaps over the front of the hip joint.

- **Muscle Strains**: Strained hamstring muscles or groin pulls can cause hip pain, while surrounding strained muscles and muscle spasms of the hip can contribute to hip pain.

- **Hip Fractures**: Osteoporosis patients and the elderly can experience hip fractures. Surgical procedures are required to mend this condition.

- **Stress Fractures**: High impact sports are common causes for stress fractures.

- **Pelvis Ligaments and Tendons**: Improperly healed ligaments or ligaments that have been overstretched cannot properly support the hip joint causing intense joint pain. Tendons that may be torn at the bone will cause lack of support for the hip joint causing intense pain as well.

Treatment Options

Natural—Non-Surgical Procedures

- Stem Cell/PRP (platelet rich plasma) injections
- Regenerative Orthopedics (Prolotherapy) injections
- Chinese herbal medicine and herbal patches
- Rest
- Ice and heat therapy
- Ultrasound
- Chiropractic care

Medical—Non-Surgical Procedures

- Non-steroidal anti-inflammatory drugs (NSAIDS)
- Pain and anti-inflammatory medications

Medical—Surgical Procedures (only when all else fails)

- Total hip replacement
- Partial hip replacement

FRACTURES

Fractures are spinal bones that are not completely cracked through such as a break. They usually are surface cracks that can occur by a fall, accident, or trauma. They are common in osteoporosis patients who experience minimal traumas or falls.

Symptoms

- Pain

- Instability of balance

Root Causes

- Falls, trauma, accidents

Treatment Options

Natural—Non-Surgical Procedures

- Physical therapy
- Stem Cell/PRP (platelet-rich plasma) injections
- Regenerative Orthopedics (Prolotherapy) injections
- Chinese herbal medicine and herbal patches
- Rest and use of bracing
- Food selection based on blood type

Medical—Non-Surgical Procedures

- Pain medications
- Spinal Epidural, Cortisone injections

Medical—Surgical Procedure (only when all else fails)

- Bone grafting

TENNIS ELBOW INJURY

The inflammation of the tendons of the elbow usually on the outer side of the elbow joint is referred to as lateral epicondylitis.

Symptoms

- Very painful condition; pain radiating from elbow into the forearm and wrist

Root Causes

- Sports: tennis, poor technique; golf
- Repetitive use: commercial painters, construction workers such as plumbers

- Excessive use: culinary motions like continually cutting veggies and meats

Treatment Options

Natural—Non-Surgical Procedures

- Stem cell/PRP (platelet rich plasma) injections
- Regenerative Orthopedics (Prolotherapy) injections
- Exercise
- Rest
- Physical therapy
- Chinese herbal medicine and herbal patches

Medical—Non-Surgical Procedures

- Non-steroidal anti-inflammatory drugs (NSAIDS)

Medical—Surgical Procedures (only when all else fails)

- Surgery

WHIPLASH INJURY

Whiplash injury is a soft tissue injury. It affects the ligaments and muscles in the back of the neck.

Symptoms

- Very painful condition in the back of your neck
- Muscle spasms
- Neck stiffness

Root Causes

- The most common cause is from rear-end automobile collisions.
- A sudden hyperextension movement (head being whipped backward) followed by hyper flexion of the neck (head being whipped forward)

Treatment Options

Natural—Non-Surgical Procedures

- Soft foam cervical collar (for stability)
- Physical therapy exercises for reducing pain, stiffness, and regaining function
- Chinese herbal medicine and herbal patches
- Acupuncture
- Stem cell/PRP (platelet rich plasma) injections
- Regenerative Orthopedics (Prolotherapy) injections
- Chiropractic care

Medical—Non-Surgical Procedures

- Non-steroidal anti-inflammatory drugs (NSAIDS)

ROTATOR CUFF INJURY

When the tendons of the shoulder joint (ball and socket) area are painfully inflamed, irritated, and swollen, this condition is referred to as Rotator Cuff Tendonitis (RCT). RCT affects men and women of all ages.

Symptoms

- Painful when moving the shoulder upward, outward, or across the body
- Painful when sleeping, difficult pulling the covers over the body, lying on bad shoulder
- All overhead lifting or working by raising the shoulders is painful

Root Causes

- Many sports activities with repetitive movements: overhead rotation, pitching motion in baseball, lifting and/or pressing weights overhead, swimming

- Career/Hobby: golf swing, construction worker, painter
- Chronic inflammation (months) can induce tears of the tendon tissue
- Age-related: 40-plus group, weekend warriors repetitiously throwing football, baseball

Treatment Options

Natural—Non-Surgical Procedure

- Chinese herbal medicine and herbal patches
- Stem Cell/PRP (platelet rich plasma) injections
- Regenerative Orthopedics (Prolotherapy) injections
- Ice packing on shoulder
- Physical therapy
- Chiropractic care
- Rest
- Avoiding activities that irritate the shoulders

Medical—Non-Surgical Procedures

- Non-steroidal anti-inflammatory drugs (NSAIDS)
- Cortisone Steroid injections

Medical Surgical Procedures (only when all else fails)

- Surgery

TORN MENISCUS (KNEE) INJURY

Torn meniscus is when the C-shaped pieces of cartilage around the knee are injured. The actual cartilage tissue that is very fibrous becomes frayed like a rope that starts tearing apart. This condition can be extremely painful causing temporary disability and dysfunctional movement at the knee joint, particularly because it is a weight-bearing joint.

Symptoms

- Painful when turning or twisting
- Very stiff
- Swelling
- Popping sounds due to swollen tissue
- Difficulty straightening the knee

Root Causes

- Sudden twisting or exertion or start and stop motions
- Long periods of kneeling, squatting, and poor position when lifting
- Athletics: torn meniscus can accompany an anterior cruciate ligament injury causing tremendous swelling, inflammation, and pain

Treatment Options

Natural—Non-Surgical Procedures

- Rest; avoid any activity or movement that would irritate the knee joint
- Ice; reduces swollen tissue and reduces pain; inflammation = pain
- Stem Cell/PRP (platelet rich plasma) injections
- Regenerative Orthopedics (Prolotherapy) injections
- Chinese herbal medical and herbal patches
- Exercise: physical therapy to strengthen surrounding muscles of the knee to stabilize the knee joint

Medical—Non-Surgical Procedures

- Medication: Non-steroidal anti-inflammatory drugs reduce inflammation and ease pain

- Orthotics: arch support for balanced weight distribution

Medical — Surgical Procedures (only after all else fails)

- Surgery

TORN LIGAMENTS

Ligaments are elastic but can be overly stretched (torn). Ligaments are fibrous dense tissue that strengthens and stabilizes all joints. Ligaments connect bone to bone.

Symptoms

- Usually a snapping or cracking sound
- Pain
- Painful bruising and swelling

Root Causes

- Overstretching
- Hyperlaxity, double-jointed = over-stretching the ligament
- An untreated ligament will lead to joint instability and eventually lead to cartilage wear and possibly osteoarthritis.

Treatment Options

Natural—Non-Surgical Procedures

- Stem Cell/PRP (platelet rich plasma) injections
- Regenerative Orthopedics (Prolotherapy) injections
- Chinese herbal medicine and herbal patches

Medical—Surgical Procedures (only when all else fails)

- Surgery

TENDON TEAR

Tendons are fibrous tissue that attach muscle to bone. When injured it is referred to as a tear. Tendon injuries are classified on a sliding scale of 1st, 2nd and 3rd degree strains.

Symptoms

- **First degree strain**: Pain and discomfort; easiest to heal or rehabilitate

- **Second degree strain**: Major pain, discoloration, and swelling

- **Third degree strain**: Complete tear, joint instability, and muscle dysfunction

Root Causes

- Injuries to tendons usually occur when involving joints that move in more than one direction: ankles, wrists, shoulders, and hips.

Treatment Options

Natural—Non-Surgical Procedures

- First degree strain: Rest, Ice, Compression, Elevate (RICE)

- Second degree strain: Rest, Ice, Compression, Elevate (RICE)

- Stem Cell/PRP (platelet rich plasma) injections

- Regenerative Orthopedics (injections)

- Chinese herbal medicine and herbal patches

- Food selections based on blood type

Medical—Non-Surgical Procedures

- Second degree strain: Anti-inflammatory medications, analgesics, RICE

Medical—Surgical Procedure (only when all else fails)

- Third degree strain: surgical repair; lengthy rehabilitation

Note: Thorough stretching and strengthening of surrounding muscles for increased range of motion (ROM) of a joint will prevent possible tendon injury.

TENDONITIS

Irritation or inflammation of a tendon is referred to as tendonitis. This condition affects any one of the fibrous cords that attach the bone to muscle. Tendonitis can occur in any joint of the body, but usually occurs in the shoulders, elbows, wrists, ankles, and hips. Overuse or repetitive use is generally the cause in many types of sports: tennis (elbow), swimming (shoulders), golf (elbow), baseball pitchers (shoulders), even track and field jumpers (knees).

Symptoms (at the attachment of the tendon at the bone)

- A dull pain
- Tenderness
- Mild swelling

Root Causes

- Overuse; through repetition over time
- Explosive injury, extreme force of the joint
- Irritation of a weakened tendon

Treatment Options

Natural—Non-Surgical Procedures

- Stem Cell/PRP (platelet rich plasma) injections
- Regenerative Orthopedics (Prolotherapy) injections
- Chinese herbal medicine and herbal patches
- Rest and icing

- Food selection based on blood type
- Exercises; stretches and strengthening joint and surrounding muscles

Medical—Non-Surgical Procedures

- Non-steroidal anti-inflammatory drugs (NSAIDs)
- Corticosteroid injections to reduce inflammation can be damaging to the tendon with repeated injections potentially weakening and leading to a tendon rupture

CARPAL TUNNEL SYNDROME

Carpal tunnel is a narrow, rigid passageway of ligaments and bones at the base of the hand. It houses the median nerve and tendons that run down from the forearm. Carpal Tunnel Syndrome is when the median nerve gets pressed or squeezed at the wrist and becomes irritated and/or inflamed. This condition becomes very painful.

Symptoms

- Gradual burning sensation, tingling and/or itching in palm of hand, fingers, thumb, index and middle fingers

Root Causes

- Trauma or injury to the wrist, swelling
- Sprain or fracture, swelling and pain
- Overactive pituitary gland, water retention during pregnancy, RA, joint stress

Treatment Options
Natural—Non-Surgical Procedures

- Rest, immobilize the wrist
- Ice packs

- Natural diuretics, Vitamin B6
- Stem Cell/PRP (platelet rich plasma) injections
- Regenerative Orthopedics (Prolotherapy) injections
- Chinese herbal medicine and herbal patches

Medical—Non-Surgical Procedures

- Non-steroidal anti-inflammatory drugs (NSAIDs)
- Medication, anti-inflammatory
- Orally administered diuretics
- Corticosteroid injections

Medical—Surgical Procedures (only when all else fails)

- Surgery

SPRAIN

A sprain is a stretch and/or tear of a ligament, the fibrous band of connective tissue that joins the end of one bone with another. Ligaments stabilize and support the body's joints. There are three levels of sprain severity:

- Severe sprain causes excruciating pain at the moment of injury. This is when the ligament actually tears completely from the bone. This causes a nonfunctional joint.

- Moderate sprain produces a partial tear of the ligament. This condition contributes to instability and swelling of the joint.

- Mild sprain causes a stretched ligament, but the joint remains stabilized.

Symptoms

- Inflammation, pain, swelling and bruising
- Categories; mild, moderate and severe
- Popping or snapping sound

Root Causes

A sprain is caused directly or indirectly by a fall or hit to the body, a trauma, etc. The trauma can be such that it that knocks a joint out of position, overstretches, and, in severe cases, ruptures the supporting ligaments. Typically this injury occurs when an individual turns the ankle while playing sports, running, stepping on uneven surfaces, or maybe lands wrong on an outstretched arm, etc. Anybody is susceptible to a sprain—from athletes to people who are overweight and in poor condition.

Treatments Options

Natural—Non-Surgical Procedures

- Stem cell/PRP (platelet rich plasma) injections
- Regenerative Orthopedics (Prolotherapy) injections
- Rest, ice, compression, and elevation (RICE)

Medical—Non-Surgical Procedures

- Mild condition — medical doctor evaluation of the injury to establish treatment and rehabilitation plan
- Severe sprain — may require surgery or immobilization followed by months of therapy

STRAIN

A strain is an injury of a muscle and/or tendon. Tendons are fibrous cords of tissue that attach muscles to bone. There are three levels or stages of a strain:

- Severe strains — partially or full rupture of a muscle and/or tendon. This leaves the individual incapacitated. Acute strains — are caused by a direct hit to the body, overstretching, or excessive muscle contraction.
- Moderate strains — Loss of some muscle function where the torn muscle/tendon has been overstretched.

- Mild strain — a slight muscle/tendon stretched or pulled.

Symptoms

- Pain
- Muscle spasm and weakness
- Swelling, inflammation
- Cramping

Root Causes

Chronic strains are the result of overuse (prolonged, repetitive movement) of muscles and tendons. Inadequate rest breaks during intensive training precipitates a strain. Anybody is susceptible to a strain, from athletes to people who are overweight and in poor condition.

Treatment Options

Natural—Non-Surgical Procedures

- Stem cell/PRP (platelet rich plasma) injections
- Regenerative Orthopedics (Prolotherapy) injections
- Rest, ice, compression, and elevation (RICE)

Medical—Non-Surgical Procedures

- Mild strain — medical doctor evaluation of the injury to establish treatment and rehabilitation plan
- Severe strain — may require surgery or immobilization followed by months of therapy

Note: Reduce Your Risk of Injury

- Exercise to build muscle strength
- Stretch daily
- Wear properly fitting shoes
- Eat for your blood type
- Warm up before sports or recreational activities

MUSCLE SPASM/MUSCLE CRAMP

Muscle spasm, charley horse, or muscle cramp as they are called, can happen at any time unexpectedly. The muscle spasm is when the muscle in the calf, thigh, foot, arms, etc., suddenly becomes rock hard and very tight.

Symptoms

- Extreme pain
- Very tight muscle

Root Causes

- Dehydration
- Poor blood circulation
- Muscle fatigue, exercising in the heat
- Nutrient deficiency: magnesium, potassium, and calcium
- Insufficient stretching and overexertion of the calf muscle
- Side effects from medications

Treatment Options

Natural—Non-Surgical Procedures

- Massaging and stretching the muscle
- Icing the muscle or warming the muscle; Epsom bath or Jacuzzi

Medical—Non-Surgical Procedures

- None

Note: If you frequently experience cramps or spasms for no apparent reason, you should speak to your doctor, as they could signal a medical problem that requires treatment.

BONE SPURS

Bone spurs are also referred to as osteophytes, which are projections of the body's normal bone structure. Common sites for bone spurs are hips, knees, spine, hands, shoulders, and feet. When this calcification grows and touches or presses on other tissue or nerves, it can be very painful.

Symptoms

- Numbness, pain, and tenderness
- Painful spots on the feet or heels when pressure from body weight is applied
- Some spurs, if located in a joint, can disrupt normal joint function

Root Causes

- Tendonitis, Osteoarthritis, aging process
- Pain in the spine or feet
- Break up of soft tissue that covers the ends of the bone

Treatment Options

Natural—Non-Surgical Procedures

- Weight loss to lessen the pressure on the painful area
- Ice therapy
- Rest
- Food selections based on blood type
- Lack of trace minerals (see Resources)

Medical—Non-Surgical Procedures

- Medications
- Cortisone injections

Medical — Surgical Procedures

- Surgery; see Chart A

SECTION IV

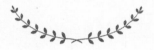

TREATMENT OPTIONS

CHAPTER 8

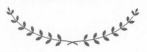

ADULT STEM CELL TREATMENTS

*"Your own stem cells —the new frontier in
alternative medicine!"* —DR. JOE

I chose to separate adult stem cell treatment from the following Glossary of Treatments so I could share my personal experiences with this technology and the immediate results I experienced which saved me from a premature surgery. Adult stem cell treatments are the perfect remedy for people who have musculoskeletal problems and conditions. Today, there are many more forms of treatments and technology available than what was common or popular even 25 years. Even as I write this book, I am still in pursuit of finding more remedies, protocols, modalities, etc., that help individuals as yourself find that right remedy or combination of procedures that will relieve or eliminate chronic pain so you can return to a pain-free life as it was meant to be enjoyed.

Stem cell treatments are all-natural treatments that are very beneficial for hip, knee, shoulder, and most every joint including back problems, like stenosis, etc. Stem cells actually heal and/or grow new cartilage tissue in the joint and surrounding soft tissue and reduce the pain level dramatically. The beauty is stem cell treatments can prevent unnecessary knee, hip, shoulder, or back surgeries. In my opinion the most effective treatments are stem cell and PRP along with regenerative orthopedics (listed in the Glossary). I strongly recommend these treatments first for a damaged joint before opting for replacement surgery.

I have personally had stem cell and PRP treatments done on my lower back and cervical spine (neck) with fantastic results. After trying every type of therapy for years in hopes of relieving the pain in my lower back, I came in contact with a doctor who specialized in arthritic and injury pain in 2008. I had been dealing with crippling back pain for several years prior and knew my back was in serious trouble.

It was a totally new experience for me. The fascinating thing about stem cell therapy is the "medicine," as Dr. Farschian calls it, is my own stem cells and blood components that he injected into my lower back and joints.

That first stem cell injection treatment was in September 2008. He suggested I see him in November to determine whether I required a second treatment. When November rolled around, Lori and I were busy with family and business. I noticed that I wasn't having much if any pain in my lower back, so I didn't feel the need for a second treatment.

In February of the next year, I felt daily back pain, so I scheduled a second stem cell treatment. This time it took two treatments because my back condition was complicated due to the emergency back surgery I had 20 years previously and what I was dealing with currently. As I mentioned previously, after an invasive surgery the body grows scar tissue, which was invading and impinging nerves in my lower back. In addition, I had four bulging discs and moderate stenosis that were all causing sciatic pain. Each time I received a stem cell treatment, I experienced more and more relief.

Later in 2009, I experienced severe pain that ran down my left shoulder, arm, and into my hand and fingers. The pain was almost unbearable. I lost 90 percent strength in my left triceps muscle in my upper arm plus major atrophy (muscle deterioration) of that muscle. I had bulging discs in my cervical spine (neck) at the C-7, C-8, and C-9 joints of my neck. Because I already had success with the stem cell/ PRP injection treatments for my lower back, I headed back to Miami for stem cell/PRP treatments in my neck. After two treatments, within eight weeks all the pain was gone. I began strengthening my triceps muscle, and over time I regained almost all muscle size in my left arm.

One of the concerns you should have if dealing with bulging discs, pinched nerves, or any condition that involves the impingement of the nerve, is permanent nerve damage. Our nerves transport electrical energy to our organs, muscles, and other parts of our body to keep them alive and functioning normal. When a nerve is impinged or compressed, the energy force or electrical life is choked out and the organ or muscle tissue will start to prematurely die or lose its normal functionality. This is where I experienced the benefits from stem cell treatment as it strengthened the ligaments and tendons surrounding and supporting my vertebrae, which in turn relieved pressure on the disc and nerve.

I have personally spoken with men and women of all ages with all types of injuries, whether from sports, automobile accidents, falls, and even older folks who had arthritis in the knees or hips or bulging discs in their neck or back, who all were healed after having stem cell/ PRP injections.

As I mentioned before, there is a tendency for most people to gravitate to conventional medical procedures and medicine without considering other alternatives that are not mainstream medicine and especially if they sound cutting edge or out of the box. But if you are suffering daily with chronic pain and have not found the solution to your problem or are not satisfied with the way your doctor is handling your condition, then the information in this book should be very encouraging—there *is* something that can fix your problem. Again, try *everything* else first before opting for surgery.

ADULT STEM CELL THERAPY

Every human being has stem cells. Stem cells are our body's remodeling and repair crew. Adult stem cells that are the most popular in application and research in association with tissue repair are the mesenchymal stem cells. Stem cells are found in the bone marrow, blood, and adipose tissue or body fat. The greatest amount of stem cells, by the millions, are found in adipose or fat tissue.

These cells go to areas in your body like the joints, meniscus tissue, ligaments, tendons, and rotator cuff where blood and oxygen flow is limited or nonexistent—areas of hypoxia or low oxygen content. These areas do not heal on their own because the body cannot get enough repair cells to the injured area. Once injected into your body, these stem cells begin repairing and rebuilding the damaged area(s).

Because stem cells are unspecialized, they can grow new bone tissue, cartilage, organs, nerves, new breasts for a cancer reconstruction patient, and even damaged or torn muscle tissue. Adult stem cell treatments are valid and efficacious; many top professional sports athletes use stem cell treatments to rebuild and repair the injured areas of their joints so they can get back to their sport in record time. Yes, stem cell treatment is the wave of the 21st century!

Adult stem cells not only rejuvenate tissue, they can reconstruct various types of injuries and defects. Stem cell injections, or platelet injections, grow into and even multiply cartilage tissue in the joints, saving a patient from unnecessary types of medical surgical procedures like knee or hip replacements. There was the time when a bone-on-bone joint condition was next to a death sentence of the joint. Now that same joint can be rejuvenated with PRP (platelet rich plasma) and stem cells and actually have new cartilage growth providing the protection between the bones it once had when healthy. The beauty is that this procedure is all natural with no ill side effects, no dangerous additives or chemicals or medications; therefore there is no toxicity in the body, just the individual's own blood and components.

Because all individual cases are different, results will vary. It usually takes two to three months for the repair process to take place, but noticeable improvement can be experienced well before that.

Imagine being an outpatient, having a mini liposuction of the tummy, a blood draw, having your own stem cells extracted from the fat or adipose tissue and blood, go through its proper treatment so it can be injected into your damaged knee, hip, shoulder, neck, spine, wherever—all within a few hours, and then being sent home the same day. This procedure is by far the most effective I experienced—it is the wave of the future for restoring health.

For advanced stem cell treatments, natural cancer therapies and holistic healing therapies, visit our clinic ReJuv U, located in the Bahama Islands. For further information go to: Resources on page 341 in the back of the book.

STEM CELL TERMINOLOGY

- **Adult Stem Cells**—Also referred to as somatic cells; adult stem cells include any body stem cell other than an egg or sperm cell in the female or male, respectively.

- **Stem Cells**—Cells that can divide and self-renew for an indefinite period of time to differentiate into specialized cells.

- **Autologous Transfer**—Transfer of adult stem cells to a different location in the same person. The transplant of stem cells to different areas of the body carries little risk of the resulting tissue being rejected.

- **Cord Blood Stem Cells**—Stem cells present in the umbilical cord blood that can be collected after birth and stored for later use in therapeutic treatment. Cord blood stem cells are haematopoietic (they can produce blood cells), and are commonly used to treat cancer patients who have undergone chemotherapy.

- **Differentiation**—Cell differentiation is the result of the interaction between a cell's genes and the external environment including physical and chemical conditions. The cell can differentiate into specialized cells such as those of the liver, heart, or bone. Various techniques have been devised to cause a cell to differentiate into specific cell types for therapeutic purposes by influencing the signaling pathways of proteins on the cells' external surface; this is known as directed differentiation.

- **Embryonic Stem Cells**—Stem cells capable of dividing for a long period of time without differentiation. These stem cells are derived from pre-implantation embryos and have been the subject of much debate in medical bioethics. Due to their primitive (undifferentiated) nature they can lead to the creation of many cell types, which may cause problems if implanted in living tissue without careful control. Embryonic stem cell use is very controversial in many religious, societal, and cultural circles.

- **Hematopoietic Stem Cells**—These stem cells form the red and white blood cells and platelets and are found in bone marrow and umbilical cord blood.

- **Mesenchymal Stem Cells**—The current, somewhat general term for non-blood somatic (adult) stem cells from a variety of tissues in the body.

- **Multi-potent**—A stem cell can be multi-potent in that it has the ability to differentiate into a number of different cell types in the body, such as blood cells, bone cells, or cartilage.

- **Regenerative Medicine**—A general term describing the use of stem cells differentiated to form specific cell types in repairing or replacing damaged cells or tissues.

- **Somatic (adult) Stem Cells**—An increasingly used source of stem cells derived from adult tissues such as bone marrow, blood, fat, and other organs. Less potent than embryonic stem cells, somatic cells have a more limited number of cell types into which they can differentiate.

It's obvious that I highly recommend stem cell treatment because of what I have experienced, as have thousands of other people. But there are many other treatment options that you will certainly want to explore in your search to be pain-free.

The Glossary of Treatments lists several procedures that are either from a conventional medical perspective or a natural alternative perspective. Hopefully one or more of these will be of assistance to you in making the right decision for your condition. But as you look into determining what works best for your specific condition, please understand that one person's condition can be normal and uncomplicated, whereas another person's condition may be complex and require more than one type of treatment.

So don't listen to those who say they tried a certain treatment and had no results; don't get discouraged, each person responds differently because of their unique physiology.

The Glossary is not exhaustive, but it does cover many treatments that you may or may not be familiar with. Perhaps you will find one that could be the very treatment your condition needs.

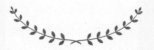

GLOSSARY OF TREATMENTS

REGENERATIVE ORTHOPEDICS

Regenerative Orthopedics is the 21st century non-surgical stem cell technology that addresses orthopedic problems and musculo-skeletal pain.

Of the following common treatments, I have saved space in the beginning of the list for this special, cutting-edge type of treatment. I believe in the efficacious results of this technology and treatment for musculoskeletal pain, etc. I can also attest to its effectiveness from firsthand experience. The following description of this technology and treatment has been presented by an associate of mine and my personal physician, Dr. Mark Walter.

WHAT IS REGENERATIVE ORTHOPEDICS?

Regenerative Orthopedics or RO is a non-surgical approach where we use small precise injections of PRP with or without stem cells to regenerate damaged joints, ligaments and tendons. The PRP (platelet rich plasma) is rich in your body's own growth factors and is spun down from a simple blood draw in a process that takes about 30 minutes.

Stem cells are typically harvested from your own abdominal fat which is lipoaspirated in a simple office-based surgical procedure. The fat is then processed to yield the stem cell injectate in a process that takes a couple of hours. It should be noted that in all of our regenerative orthopedic procedures we use only the patients' own tissues i.e. blood and fat (referred to as "autologous" tissues) so there is no foreign or unnatural tissues/products ever injected.

Once prepared, the PRP with or without stem cells is injected at the precise location of injury or degeneration and stimulates the body to "regenerate" the damaged structure. If done properly, these regenerative orthopedic injections are very safe and can yield impressive results with many orthopedic and musculoskeletal conditions.

The concept and art of regenerative injections to treat musculoskeletal conditions has actually been around for many years in a discipline called Prolotherapy. Prolo typically used injections of dextrose and other natural *proliferants* to stimulate healing. What is new are the advances in PRP and stem cell technology that allows us to more easily and reliably isolate and concentrate growth factors and stem cells and use these in properly targeted injections to help stimulate the natural healing of degenerated and/or damaged structures.

What type of conditions can RO help?

I have personally been using these regenerative injection techniques for about 15 years to treat many orthopedic conditions including osteoarthritis, ligament sprains, and tendonitis. Common conditions include OA of the knee or hip and rotator cuff tendonitis. We also commonly treat back pain and neck pain, whether due to degenerative disc problems or other causes. As for conditions such as sports injuries, wrist problems, or ankle problems, plantar fasciitis, tennis elbow, and whiplash injuries I consider that in many cases the regenerative approach is by far the most effective treatment option.

It should be noted that in RO we often have a very different diagnosis as to what the "primary pain generator" is. In our view joint capsules, ligaments, and tendons are far bigger pain generators than bone, cartilage, or true nerve impingement. For example, an MRI might very well show disc abnormalities in a patient with back pain but this does not mean that it is the primary cause of the pain. A very common scenario is that the patient has a pelvic strain (that was not diagnosed!) causing the pain and incidentally happens to have degenerated or damaged discs. Unfortunately, MRI (and x-rays of course) have very limited application to correct diagnosis of the primary "pain generators," as even MRI misses the subtle sprains and strains that are so often the true root cause of the pain.

This begs the question of how can we accurately diagnose the cause of a problem? Ultrasound can be useful in certain situations but by far the most important diagnostic maneuver is a history and physical exam with an experienced regenerative orthopedic specialist. When I examine a patient, I directly palpate suspected structures to try and elicit the "Jump sign." If I can reproduce the patient's pain by directly palpating a specific structure (ligament compression test), I am confident that I have identified the correct pain generator. This is where the patient requires the regenerative injections.

In most cases it may take several treatments sessions to achieve optimal results, usually spaced two to four weeks apart. Overall, if I examine a patient and can identify the particular structures that are damaged with a positive "jump sign" my personal success rate is in the range of 80%.

Do you start with just PRP or PRP and stem cells?

This choice depends on several factors such as: how severe the damage is, how much time we have, the age and overall health of the patient, if the patient is a good candidate for the fat harvesting lipoaspirate procedure, financial considerations, etc. In general PRP can be used successfully when it is a joint capsule, ligament, or tendon that is the primary problem. If we are dealing with lots of cartilage loss and severe degeneration, a chronic burned-out case, then stem cells should be considered to give us the best chance at successful joint regeneration. In this case, PRP is also added as a fertilizer to help the stem cells grow, proliferate, and repair the damaged structures. If the patient has a stem cell treatment and still has significant symptoms four weeks after treatment, I usually recommend a PRP booster to reignite the stem cell healing.

A Regenerative Orthopedic doctor should be a specialist!

The beauty of the RO approach is that it is safe, minimally invasive, and can yield some pretty spectacular results; *however*, the effectiveness (and safety) of the procedure is totally dependent on the expertise of the specialist you choose, as well as the quality of the PRP and stem cells used. My recommendation is that you try and find a medical doctor who is well trained and experienced in regenerative injections and is also advanced in PRP and stem cell preparation. As far as diagnostic/injection skills, I would look for a doc who has been doing regenerative injections/Prolotherapy for a long time and had specific training in regenerative injections. I consider Regenerative Orthopedics as a specialty onto itself and for optimal results I would suggest choosing a doc who is fully dedicated to the specialty.[1]

Note: Dr. Walter is a pioneer in the field of Regenerative Orthopedics. He is McGill trained (1980) and has a background in family practice and sports medicine. Dr. Walter has made regenerative orthopedic injections his full-time practice for 15 years and has worked with some of the top prolotherapy teachers in the world. Dr. Walter is a member of the American Academy of Orthopedic Medicine and has lectured extensively about the regenerative injection approach.

ACUPUNCTURE

"I cannot see a better solution to long-term chronic pain. There is no question in my mind that acupuncture is safer than surgery or drugs." —DR. BRUCE POMERANZ, Neuroscientist, University of Toronto

Acupuncture is a time-tested, safe, effective, natural, and drug-free way to eliminate pain. Unlike other methods of handling pain, there are no side effects. Well-known and leading national and international health organizations acknowledge the benefits of acupuncture in treating and eliminating pain due to a wide range of causes.

Acupuncture practitioners recognize there is a vital energy that flows or circulates throughout the body. This flow of vital energy, or what is referred to as Qi (pronounced "chee"), circulates through a series of pathways called meridians. Meridians transport life-giving energy and nourishment to every cell, tissue, organ, and gland in the body.

Blockage or something that impedes the flow of nourishment and energy throughout the body is when an individual can experience illness or painful conditions. Energy flow can be blocked due to physical trauma, poor diet, emotional trauma, and chemical, physical, and emotional stress.

Acupuncture is performed by inserting fine, sterile needles at specific points into the body. From there the practitioner can break up the blockages of energy flow to various organs, muscles, tissues, and glands and help restore their natural function. In turn, pain is relieved and the individual can enjoy pain-free living. Acupuncture works well in weight loss and fibromyalgia patients.

My experience with acupuncture goes back to 1975 when I traveled to Toronto, Canada, from Buffalo, New York for back and shoulder treatments. My shoulder had bothered me for years from competitive weight training, and after just one acupuncture treatment the pain was gone. Please keep in mind the fact that we are all different, we all respond differently and at different paces to this and any treatment.

MYOFASCIAL RELEASE MASSAGE (MRM)

Due to stored up stress and tension in your muscles, ligaments, and tendons (connective tissue) these tissues become stiff and somewhat immoveable, which results in discomfort, or even pain, in your everyday life. MRM relieves this discomfort through stretches.

A MRM singular can identify the trouble areas in your body by running their fingers or palpating until they hit a painful spot through a massage. Then, stretches are used to open the muscles and connective tissues that are holding the stress. The massage focuses deeply on ligature as well as muscles. The stretches can be intense at times so it is important to communicate with the therapist how you are feeling throughout the massage session and also a day or two later.

When the fascia or connective tissue tightens or gets tight, it causes a restriction of muscle and other tissues. This can result in back pain and loss of motion. Injuries, stress, inflammation, trauma, and poor posture supposedly contribute to this tightness. Individuals who have been involved in an auto accident, have had a joint injury, or are stressed out to the max can benefit from this form of massage. Ultimately, the adhesive or "tissue-lock" that is restricting muscle and joint movement is released and then tension, stress, and pain are alleviated. I have personally found that this deep tissue massage and stretch has allowed my joints and muscle motion to improve, allowing me to be more flexible, and at the same time less painful.

For individuals suffering from fibromyalgia, back pain, and other muscle-associated health issues, MRM can help. This therapy has also been used to treat pains of a different kind, including those associated with chronic fatigue, severe tension, and anxiety. It has even been used as therapy for repetitive stress injuries of the muscular-skeletal system.

MRM loosens and frees muscle and connective tissue. This means that any physical condition where there is tightness of the fascia, MRM can relieve it. MRM handles a myriad of conditions such as muscular and joint pains, fatigue, tensions, and even some of the physical side effects of old age. It is also thought to help with injuries and other sustained physical damage.

PERSONAL ILLNESS PROFILE (PIP)

"To rid your body of disease and illness you must eradicate the root cause—not treat the symptoms." —DR. JOE

PIP is an extensive health evaluation that includes all ten body systems* through saliva testing. The evaluation exposes which system in your body is compromised and by what root cause. Some of these root causes can be anything from a parasite such as mold, fungus, slime mold, worms, or environmental toxins such as chlorine, dyes, or other solvents. Other root causes may be food allergies or hormonal imbalances.

Dr. Robert Christiano, ND, who specializes in electro-magnetic medicine, explains that, "PIP primarily functions through frequency or is a frequency treatment." Frequency treatment can be applied through a contact device (hand-held metal probes). If a person has very thick, calloused hands and feet, frequencies can be applied using plasma light. Plasma light frequencies penetrate very deeply into the body.

All matter has an electro-magnetic frequency attached to it. This frequency is achieved by millions of elements (periodic table of elements) colliding into each other. This causes a vibration that creates a frequency.

So how does frequency treatment work?

Dr. Bob from www.newwavewellness.com says, "Keeping it simple, let's take the pinworm. A pinworm, which infests the intestinal tract, carries with it the frequencies of: 422 hz, 423 hz, 732 hz, and 4412 hz. By applying these same frequencies to the body through a contact device or through plasma light therapy, we are actually pulling the teeth out of the pinworm or negating the pinworm."

One of the greatest features of this concept is a patient can be treated long distance. By submitting a saliva sample from the PIP kit you receive, simply mail it back to Dr. Bob's office and he can do the work from there. After his diagnosis is completed, a 1-hour phone consultation is scheduled to review the results of your test, answer all of your questions, and make suggestions of what you need to kill the root cause and heal your body.

The concept is similar to "like cures like." If a person gets bitten by a snake, in many cases, the exact same snake venom will be administered to the person. Both venoms carry the same frequency, thus negating the affects. Another example: If we get grease on our hands, just plain water will not cut the grease. So we use soap. Soap is a form of grease. Carrying the same frequencies of grease, the soap cuts the grease. Another example is the opera singer who shatters glass with her voice. When that note is hit and reaches the exact frequency of glass, the glass shatters. By the way, homeopathic remedies work the same way. Also, let us not forget that *words and emotions* carry their own frequencies.

*The ten body systems are: Circulatory System, Digestive System, Intestinal System, Glandular System, Immune System, Nervous System, Reproductive System, Respiratory System, Structural System, Urinary System, plus Hormone Imbalances, Food Allergies, Parasite Infestation and Toxicity/Autointoxication.

Note: Visit my website at: www.bodyredesigning.com or call 1-800-259-2639 for more information about PIP (personal illness profile), and scheduling an appointment.

TRANSDERMAL PATCHES AND HERBAL REMEDIES

As a virtual physician with Wei Laboratories, our approach to healing acute and chronic injuries—muscle, ligament, tendon, and bone injuries, most musculoskeletal conditions, fibromyalgia, liver and gallbladder conditions, and the like—is using Chinese medicine and herbal remedies. Additional conditions we treat are with the respiratory system, MS, allergies, gluten intolerance, Shingles, Acid Reflux, etc.

Healing times are greatly reduced due to the catalyst properties of the herbal patches that take special herbal formulas deep into the body. This approach to healing involves Chinese herbal remedies including herbal juices and supplements.

The patches deliver micro-nutrition and create micro-circulation causing the body's blood flow to be greatly enhanced particularly in areas where blood flow is absent such as the very fibrous ligaments and tendons. This treatment supports the healing process that in turn allows the patient to return to normal pain-free living. This approach to eliminating pain and healing your body focuses on eradicating the "root causes" to your painful condition.

Because of the harmful and damaging side effects from pain and anti-inflammatory medications that take place in the liver, kidneys, and stomach, there are herbal juice and capsule formulas that are specifically formulated to heal and restore damaged tissue of these glands and organs and help them return to normal function—naturally!

Note: To schedule personal consultations with Dr. Joe for evaluations and remedies for your painful condition please call 1-800-259-2639.

CHIROPRACTIC CARE

Chiropractic care is often used to treat painful conditions including but not limited to back, neck, joints of the arms and legs, and headaches. It is also referred to as neuro-musculoskeletal care. Chiropractic care is a drug-free, hands-on approach to healthcare that includes patient examination, diagnosis, and treatment.

A chiropractic doctor is a healthcare professional who focuses on conditions and disorders of the musculoskeletal system and the nervous system, and the effects of these conditions and disorders on general health. Chiropractors have broad diagnostic skills and are also trained to recommend therapeutic and rehabilitative exercises, as well as to provide nutritional, dietary, and lifestyle counseling.

A good friend of mine and author of *Blueprint to Optimal Health*, Martin Monahan DC, NMD, from Saint Augustine, Florida, states that, "Pain is a double-edge sword, an unfortunate necessary evil that needs to be minimized to insure an improved quality of life. If pain is too great, it can be unbearable; if too little or masked, it can cause further pain and damage."

Assessment of patients is done through clinical examination, laboratory testing, diagnostic imaging, and other diagnostic interventions to determine when and if chiropractic treatment is appropriate.

With chiropractic care and the medical technologies of the 21st century, people can experience regenerated joints and ramped-up anti-inflammation pathways in the body, along with providing hormones and micro/macro balance to give the body the raw material to rebuild itself.

HEAT AND ICE THERAPY

The two most common types of noninvasive and nonaddictive pain-relief therapies for muscle and joint pain are the hot and cold therapies. Depending on whether the pain is new or recurring will determine whether you use cold or heat therapy.

When to Use Hot and Cold Therapy

Treat a reoccurring injury with heat. This therapy brings blood to the area and promotes healing. Most new injures cause inflammation and possibly swelling. Ice or cold therapy decreases the blood flow to the injury, thereby decreasing inflammation and swelling.

Heat Therapy

Heat opens blood vessels, which increases blood flow, supplies oxygen and nutrients to reduce pain in joints and relax sore muscles, ligaments, and tendons. Heat decreases muscle spasms and can increase range of motion. Applying superficial heat to your body can improve the flexibility of tendons and ligaments, reduce muscle spasms, and alleviate pain.

Heat therapy can be applied by an electric or microwavable heating pad, hot water bottle, gel packs, or hot water baths. The heat should be warm, not too hot, and should be maintained at a consistent temperature, if possible.

Apply heat therapy when you have stiff joints or chronic muscle and joint pain.

Proper Heat Therapy Usage

- Wrap the heating device in a thin towel.
- Apply heat for 20 minutes.
- Avoid if there's swelling (use cold first then use heat), if you have poor circulation, diabetes, or on an open wound or stitches.

- Avoid when sleeping (possible skin burn).

Cold Therapy

Cold therapy slows down blood flow to an injury, thereby reducing pain and swelling. Cold therapy slows circulation, reducing inflammation, muscle spasm, and pain. It should be used if the area is swollen or bruised.

Cold therapy is applied by an ice or gel pack.

- For the first 24 to 48 hours after an injury is sustained
- For sprains, strains, bumps, and bruises

Proper Cold Therapy Usage

- Wrap ice or ice packs in a thin towel before applying.
- Apply cold packs or ice bags to injured areas for 20 minutes.
- Remove for 10 minutes.
- Repeat; reapply several times throughout the day.

APITHERAPY

Bee Venom Therapy

I know this may sound farfetched, but the venom from the honey bee is the perfect antidote for multiple sclerosis (MS), rheumatoid arthritis, osteoarthritis, and arthritis. This treatment for chronic arthritic pain has been around for thousands of years, dating back to the ancient days and found in ancient Greek and Egypt medical writings. This treatment is popular in Eastern Europe, Asia, and South America.

There are over 40 ingredients in bee venom; one is melittin, an anti-inflammatory agent found in the venom and is many times stronger than cortisone. Bee venom also contains a substance known as adolapin, which is both anti-inflammatory and pain blocking.

Practitioners believe all the ingredients in bee venom work together to cause the body to release more natural healing compounds in its own defense. Bee venom is also said to increase blood circulation and reduce swelling.

I have personally spoken with people who have tried bee venom therapy and had great success and are pain-free. If you are suffering from chronic pain, perhaps desperation calls and you will try anything to get rid of the pain.

Should you consider bee venom therapy from your local honey beekeeper, first be tested to make sure you are not allergic to bee venom. Bee venom therapy works great for most arthritic conditions but also for RA (rheumatoid arthritis).

CHAPTER 9

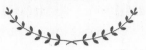

MEDICATIONS

"Prescription pain pills are the medical community's oral bandages." —Dr. Joe

Let me preface what I am about to say regarding medications. I believe there is a place for prescription medications—after all natural remedies and modalities have been exhausted or when there is an emergency situation. For example, if I get hit by a passing bus, please do not offer me some vitamin C chewable tablets—call the paramedics!

With all the good that some medications can do, the best they can do is address symptoms such as relieving pain, reducing inflammation, and the like—a medical formula for taking oral bandages—but never a cure. They are nothing more than a means to stomp out symptoms. "But let's face it," you may say, "if I'm in pain and one of these pain pills takes away my pain, I want one." Understandably so, I would too; but popping doctor's little helpers over a long period of time causes things to change—not always for the better.

What is most concerning to me about taking medications for chronic pain and inflammation are the side effects that can destroy a person's health, create additional health problems, including premature death, and the potential for drug addiction. Not a very encouraging treatment for an individual who has been injured or suffers from chronic pain.

I am certain that you know someone, in your own family or a friend's family, who has a drug addiction. I do; drug abuse has struck members in my family. It is a terrible, terrible atrocity affecting the entire family. The path of destruction seems endless when someone becomes addicted to pain medication, especially those originally designed to reduce pain from a true physiological condition but turned into a psychological and physiological dependency, a nightmare that doesn't go away.

I have spoken to many who are addicted to prescription pain medication and have heard the horror stories of financial loss, marriage and family break-ups, the numbing reality of good and decent people becoming thieves who robbed their own parents to buy more medication, plus the advancement of premature aging and related illnesses. For all these reasons and more, I chose to list some statistics from the American Academy of Pain so you, or someone you know, can make an informed decision about taking prescription pain pills.

CDC Analysis: Vital Signs: Overdoses of Prescription Opioid Pain Relievers; United States, 1999-2008[1]

Overdose deaths involving opioid pain relievers (OPR), also known as opioid analgesics, have increased and now exceed deaths involving heroin and cocaine combined.

- Prescription painkiller overdoses killed nearly 15,000 people in the US in 2008. This is more than 3 times the 4,000 people killed by these drugs in 1999.

- In 2010, about 12 million Americans (age 12 or older) reported non-medical use of prescription painkillers in the past year.

- One in 20 people in the United States, ages 12 and older, used prescription painkillers non-medically (without a prescription or just for the "high" they cause) in 2010.

- Nearly half a million emergency department visits in 2009 were due to people misusing or abusing prescription painkillers.

- Sales of OPR quadrupled between 1999 and 2010. Enough OPR were prescribed last year to medicate every American adult with a standard pain treatment dose of 5 mg of hydrocodone (Vicodin and others) taken every 4 hours for a month.

- Non-medical use of prescription painkillers costs health insurers up to $72.5 billion annually in direct healthcare costs.

- Certain groups are more likely to abuse or overdose on prescription painkillers:

- Many more men than women die of overdoses from prescription painkillers.

- Middle-aged adults have the highest prescription painkiller overdose rates.

- People in rural counties are about two times as likely to overdose on prescription painkillers as people in big cities.

- Whites and American Indian or Alaska Natives are more likely to overdose on prescription painkillers.

- About 1 in 10 American Indian or Alaska Natives age 12 or older used prescription painkillers for non-medical reasons in the past year, compared to 1 in 20 whites and 1 in 30 blacks.

- Some states have a bigger problem with prescription painkillers than others:

- Prescription painkiller sales per person were more than 3 times higher in Florida (which has the highest rate) than in Illinois (which has the lowest rate).

- In 2008/2009, non-medical use of painkillers in the past year ranged from 1 in 12 people (age 12 or older) in Oklahoma to 1 in 30 in Nebraska.

- States with higher sales per person and more non-medical use of prescription painkillers tend to have more deaths from drug overdoses.

It is not a pretty picture when we see these kinds of facts. But when multiple millions of Americans are living with chronic pain, it only stands to reason these horrifying realities exist; and if nothing is done , they will continue to exist but in greater numbers.

It stands to reason that we need to be better educated about this issue so we can be prepared and have full understanding of the pros and cons when faced with the decision of taking prescription pain pills for chronic painful conditions.

In addition to being better educated, we should be willing to make healthy lifestyle changes a priority. Thereby our healthier bodies will be more resilient to injuries, sickness and disease, plus the aging process. Healthy lifestyle changes strengthen our immune system, liver and kidneys, etc.; so if we have to be on medications, we will be fortified to stay strong and healthy.

We have been given only one body and one life to live here on planet Earth and it behooves us to do all we can as faithful stewards to remain in the best physical condition possible.

In saying all that, now we move on to the 8 Simple Steps so you can be best prepared for the worst health conditions that may come your way—and at the same time be more resilient and strengthened so you can live beyond your chronic pain!

SECTION V

8 SIMPLE STEPS TO A PAIN-FREE AND HEALTHY LIFE

STEP 1

OVERCOMING PAIN

CHAPTER 10

THE RIGHT ATTITUDE

"Focus on the purpose not the task." —Dr. Joe

In this first healthy lifestyle step, I want to talk about the importance of your attitude. The role your attitude plays is crucial; in fact, a positive attitude is what will "get you through it." No matter what you are facing, the right attitude is the key for overcoming it. The underlying factor that makes all the difference in your ability to withstand, endure, and push through is your mental attitude. The strength to overcome and walk through your healing are not medications or supplements or treatments—it is your willingness to keep a positive attitude.

As you suffer with chronic pain on a day-to-day basis, it is difficult to take your mind off of the pain. In fact, pain becomes the central part of your thoughts, actions, conversations, and can become a real distraction in your job, relationships, plans, etc. What I want to do now is encourage you to remove your focus from your painful condition to where you want to be—pain-free. I want you to start visualizing living beyond your chronic pain. You will have to remind yourself several times a day to stop focusing on the pain as it flares up and stop giving attention to the obstacles and challenges you face. Rather, focus on living pain-free.

I was able to overcome a very challenging career decision in my life at an early age that taught me how to look past my painful situation and stay focused on where I wanted to go—living beyond my chronic pain. Even right up to this very moment of writing my book I strive to keep a positive attitude every day regarding all aspects of my life.

We all know how debilitating and mentally draining chronic pain can be. It will rob you of hope and a bright future. It becomes a dark looming cloud of discouragement and gloom. That is why I am encouraging you to do your best to look past the immediate obstacles and challenges that come with the territory and focus on living beyond your chronic painful condition. This positive attitude will definitely help you in making important decisions, whether it is surgery, career changes, loss of income, family issues, etc. It takes effort, but I was able to overcome many obstacles to get where I wanted to go—and you will too!

WILLING TO CHANGE!

Before I share my experience, let's talk about change. Unless you are willing to change from a lifestyle that is less than desirable when it comes to your health and embrace new and exciting lifestyle practices that can change your health and quality of life for the good, then there is no hope for you.

Change comes hard because most people have never been taught how to develop a positive attitude. This is why you see so many seminars on positive thinking for getting out of debt or how to gain wealth or how to overcome negative obstacles that prevent you from being all you can be. Most of us have a tendency to cling to what we feel good about or what makes us feel safe and comfortable. Because we are creatures of habit, change is difficult to make. But when the heat is turned up and your circumstances change, and you are facing a health crisis like crippling joint inflammation or degenerative joint disease where pain medication doesn't help and you cannot do the things you used to do, it is very easy to fall into a negative, pessimistic mindset and give up on your hopes of living pain-free.

Plan to look at your circumstance with a more positive mindset now so the new adjustments you are forced to make can be an easier transition. Our attitude is constantly bombarded when suffering from intense burning pain of sciatica or not knowing what to do when a medical treatment failed or trying to function normally in society while in pain. Any challenge that requires you to switch from the status quo to focusing on your objective or goals or purpose requires you to develop a positive attitude to be successful. The willingness to change, keeping a positive attitude and positive belief, will make all the difference in your recovery time after a surgical procedure and is a lifeline for healing and how to best manage pain.

Because your attitude is a powerful mental attribute you possess that has no boundaries or limitations, you must take time to develop it. As you read through this first healthy step, reevaluate your attitude and see if your attitude needs a positive boost to look past the challenges you are dealing with so you can focus on a life without pain.

RENEWING YOUR MIND

- Remember, you are walking through your healing!
- Be willing to change for the good!
- Look past your pain and hold on to hope!
- Focus on living beyond your chronic pain!

CHAPTER 11

THE G MAN

"Obstacles are the greatest faith builders!" —DR. JOE

Focus on the purpose not the task. That was my mantra years ago as I faced life's challenges that came my way and is something I live by today to help me get past any situations that seemingly have no solution.

At the age of 25, I had tried several different employment opportunities. I had been in the military, was attending college, and had a family of five to feed. During this time everything I did needed to be exactly planned out because my plate was more than full. I had a plan in mind to graduate with a degree in child psychology and special education. But something was stirring deep inside me, somewhat clouding my focus even though I was moving in a certain direction at the time.

My heart wanted me to be a natural health professional, a longtime love of mine. As I got in touch with my natural, God-given passion to help people be healthier, and though the prospects of being involved in natural health was very appealing to me, pulling it off was another story. There were several major obstacles to deal with, one was to relocate to Florida and another was the cost of relocating and starting a business. Sure the thoughts of palm trees, miles of sandy beaches, and the fact that Florida was not known for its snowy, ice-cold winters were pleasant dreams, but making it happen wasn't easy. My current $200 per week paycheck served as a motivator to find something more lucrative, but how could I ever take the next big step to move and make my dream come true?

LISTEN TO YOUR HEART

It all happened when I was employed by a major sanitation company in Western New York. I was the company's dealership sales rep and sold heavy-duty compactors and waste management equipment—you know, those big cardboard compactors in the back of the stores at the malls. Shortly after being with the company in that position, the company lost their dealership. I thought for sure I was going to be in the soup line, but instead I was offered the position of operations manager. Consequently, I learned how to operate a large business. And one evening my opportunity for relocating and pursuing my new career presented itself.

On a cold, wintry western New York day as the guys were finishing their garbage routes, coming back to the locker room to change clothes, punch their time cards and go home, my career change jumped out in front of me. As I was watching the guys, I noticed most of them were between 18 years of age to 25 (my age). One guy was much older; in fact, Don was 55 and looked extremely weather-beaten, tired, and weary.

I felt badly for Don and asked him how he was doing. He said he was dead tired. I asked him why he was still on the back of the G truck throwing garbage every day. He said, "When the owner of the company and I were young guys, he told me he wanted to start a sanitation company one day, and said if I would help him from the beginning that he would take good care of me." Well, Don's old friend and now owner of this huge sanitation company apparently forgot what he told Don. Consequently, Don, who was waiting for the owner to "take care of him," was instead stuck on the back of a truck. My next question for Don was, "If you could do it all over, what would you do?" He looked at me and without hesitation said, "If I were 30 years younger (that was me by the way), I would start my own garbage company, grow it, then sell it and move to where the weather is warm."

Little did Don know but his answer to my question was divine clarity for my next move. I was that 30-years-younger man he spoke about, and I knew right then what I was going to do. I would become one too—a G man!

I knew the business. I learned the ropes, but never was on the back of a truck nor ever wanted to be. This huge task that I was about to take on was not at all what my idea of making a career change was about, but it was a means to get me to my ultimate purpose. In my mind all I saw were those sandy beaches, beautiful swaying palm trees, no more snowy, ice-cold winters, and becoming a natural health professional—my vision and purpose in life!

Not coming from money nor having a cent to my name, I went to my parents to see if they would give me a loan. All I needed was $5,000 to purchase a truck to start my new business. I suppose it wasn't quite the lavish bankroll one needs for start-up money to begin a new business venture, but because I already managed a major sanitation company much larger than one man and his truck and had negotiated a pick-up contract/schedule with a homeowner association and had a check for the first month of service in advance, I figured I was as prepared as possible. My folks could see my excitement and determination and were very gracious to loan me the money; but before the conversation was over my mother said, "Just don't put your name on the truck!"

Wow! Imagine those words of encouragement? I could have easily taken to heart what my mother said and felt insulted, even defeated but I had a purpose to fulfill, so instead of giving up on my plan, I used her negative words as fuel to help motivate me for the unknown journey ahead. I knew I was in for a long haul but didn't realize exactly how long or what it would take to build this new business with hopes of one day selling it so I could move to Florida and pursue my dream.

I recall those frozen winter days when I had to wake up at 4 am, shovel my way out of the driveway, and then drive to my truck. Once there I had to start a frozen truck engine, and if I could without needing a jump, I began my day. After fighting blizzard-like conditions, freezing my fingers off climbing snow banks to get to my customers' garbage cans, and not having any flat tires or accidents, I would return home by 12 o'clock midnight. I also recall the hot summer days when the garbage smelled so terrible I could vomit. And the times when I dumped a can in the back of the truck and the soupy garbage filled with maggots splashed back in my face.

As my company grew, so did my workload and tasks. I had to remind myself many times of my purpose and goal and keep a positive attitude during those four long years. When the day-to-day tasks became overwhelming, I made myself look to the future—to where I was going, not where I was. By keeping a positive attitude and believing, I was able to accomplish more than a 25-year-old rookie entrepreneur without a penny to his name could ever have dreamed of accomplishing.

Finally I reached my goal! I sold my business and moved to Florida. Today I'm a naturopathic doctor and have owned a natural health and fitness company for the past 35 years. Oh and off the record, after growing my company for four years with several trucks seen all over town, my mother said, "Joey, you ought to put your name on the trucks so everyone will know it's you." Hmm...?

So as you face those trying times of pain, inflammation, difficulty in walking or moving without pain, worrying about your finances, or before you lose hope for your future, please remember my mantra, *focus on the purpose not the task*. You will overcome every obstacle if you are willing to change your attitude and do all that you know you should do to be pain-free and enjoy your life.

RENEWING YOUR MIND

- Focus on the purpose, *not* the task. Repeat this mantra out loud daily.

- Reinforce your attitude and thoughts that you are going to overcome!

- Look beyond all your challenges and focus on where you want to be.

- Refocus your mind from negative thoughts to positive thoughts!

- Never stop believing!

CHAPTER 12

WHEN ALL ELSE FAILS

"The bigger your God, the smaller your problem—the bigger your Problem, the smaller your God!" —DR. JOE

Developing a positive attitude is very important when facing any challenge in life. But you are going to need even more help during life's journey. I am not going to preach to you; but as one who has been down this painful road, I knew who to run to and call on for the strength I did not possess, to push through my circumstances. Whether it was those pain-ridden sleepless nights, or when my emotions were at their lowest, or just a matter of facing another pain-filled day, I needed more than a positive mental attitude to get me through. I don't know where you stand spiritually speaking but for me, prayer and dependency in my Creator and God Yahweh has ultimately proved to be the best medicine.

I can't explain or give the answers as to *why* I was not improving or why I was still in severe pain after all those times of praying for healing, but I did know that my God had a plan and purpose for this painful season of mine. It is when I leave everything in His hands that I find my greatest strength to overcome.

As a naturopathic doctor, we believe that the body has been designed in such a magnificent way that if we detoxify it, cleanse it, feed it with natural wholesome food sources and organic nutrients, keep it physically active, spend time in the natural sunlight, stay well hydrated, and think positively—the body will heal itself. This perspective is nothing new as it has been around for centuries, practiced in Chinese medicine and other ancient cultures; there are many other ancient medicinal perspectives for addressing the whole person. But when all of that has been exhausted, we still have another source of energy, strength, and power that is capable of raising the dead, healing the sick, and saving one's soul. And unless you have faced the dark thoughts of suicide because of excruciating pain or the deadly side effects of prescription pain medications, i.e., shallow breathing, it may be difficult to understand where I am coming from, unless you are one who has or is dealing with these issues and simply can't take it anymore. If that's the case, I want you to know there is good news.

Trusting in my Creator and His ways has not always come easily. Though He never actually healed me after all my prayers, He always provided comfort to my mind and heart, letting me know my destiny was in His hands and I was just to trust Him.

As a person who has always been self-dependent, self-motivated, and self-driven, I was in control most of the time. But as I found myself physically and mentally beaten down, it was those times when He became strong and I weak. People are capable of overcoming many things in their lives but when life becomes overwhelming where do you turn? For me I found peace and comfort in meditating on His Word. And it is He who will help you with your circumstances when all else fails.

As I look back through the years, having done my best to try everything else first so to dodge surgery, I have been fortunate to learn much more in terms of what options are available to people like me and you. In the process I learned more about what alternative medicine offers versus conventional medicine. I came to discover there is a variety of modalities, remedies, supplements, exercises, treatments and procedures. As a result, I have been able to take advantage of them myself and share them in this book with you. So maybe, just maybe a portion of the purpose for all I have been going through has been to be a messenger of hope to you, so you can be better equipped in finding answers to your questions, better treatment choices and options that you may not have known existed.

So as you seek the treatment or remedy to correct your problem and strive to work your way back to a pain-free life, please think about reaching out to Him, the Great Physician, as the Bible refers to Him. Should you be facing surgery or searching for the root cause to your pain and the proper treatment or procedure that will eradicate it, remember He will carry you through it. When your life is tipping the scales so to speak and you have tried everything else, remember He cares for you and will walk with you through your healing.

All that I mentioned above has to do with my desire to live a pain-free and vibrant life, again! Consider the *whole you* when you are dealing with your painful condition—remember that your thoughts are powerful and make all the difference in the outcome!

RENEWING YOUR MIND

- A positive attitude is a choice!
- Try everything else first before you opt for surgery.
- You are valuable and have worth!
- Don't allow the fear or the unknown rob you of your hope!
- Prayer is a powerful exercise for finding relief from your pain and worries.
- Trust in the Mighty One to see you through.

STEP 2

BLOOD TYPE NUTRITION—DIET

CHAPTER 13

LESS WEIGHT, LESS PAIN

"Say goodbye to painful joints—live lighter!" —Dr. Joe

As you pursue pain-free living please remember that healing, regeneration of new tissue, reduction of inflammatory pain and disease, restoration of energy levels, weight loss, etc., all start on the inside! And much of these natural changes that occur in our body, that are linked to pain-free and disease-free living, are linked to what you eat. Keep in mind that the proper food-type selections you make on a regular basis create the baseline on which to build and develop a healthier, pain-free, leaner, and more energetic and vibrant body.

Within our genetic makeup there is a genetic code for each individual. When people eat food types that match up biochemically with their genetic code—great things happen! We see a tremendous reduction in body fat when individuals make food selections based on their blood type and avoid food types that are not compatible. Not only does the individual look and feel better by losing body fat (weight), but because obesity is an inflammatory state and adipose tissue (body fat) contributes to inflammation, weight loss on its own can cause an anti-inflammatory effect, the very condition to eliminate pain. So if you are dealing with chronic inflammatory pain and disease, the first line of defense is to start making food type selections that are compatible with your blood type.

I realize that most people look to dieting to lose weight and not for the many other purposes a correct diet can provide. If you think of weight loss as the only benefit of eating correctly, it's not! Dieting off the weight is never permanent and is not a healthy lifestyle practice. But when individuals make food selections for their blood type, their eating habits become a healthy lifestyle practice for the rest of their lives. Because they are eating foods that line up with their own chemistry by which their body is fueled properly, the body will detoxify itself and create the proper environment for healing to begin, so the bodily systems can return to normal function.

When your automobile engine is full of gunk and corrosion, its performance is greatly reduced and if not attended to and serviced properly it will lose its original purpose—clean, efficient performance. The same is true when it comes to the functionality of your natural body. As your body becomes full of cellular debris, toxins, waste products, junk estrogens from petroleum products, excessive body fat tissue and inflammation, it can't function naturally, will break down, and if you don't make the proper healthy lifestyle changes, will prematurely die. The greatest difference between your automobile and your body is you can replace your automobile, but you only get one body in this lifetime.

If you are overweight and have painful knees, hips, or lower back, one of the first things you should to do is lose some weight. Just your body weight alone, as you walk or move around, causes stress and pressure on those joints; and if you are overweight, the amount of stress and pressure on the joints increases even more so. The knee joints become painful and inflamed and normal day-to-day activities become a painful struggle when carrying excess weight.

To illustrate, I'm sure you have seen or know people who are overweight and have joint problems and pain. They have difficulty walking, climbing stairs, getting around in a store, getting in and out of their vehicle. There's no doubt that their quality of life is diminished greatly and the longer they remain overweight the more damage they are doing to the joints and surrounding soft tissue like ligaments and tendons. Without individuals being aware of it, they are causing micro-tears in the soft tissue and to the cartilage in the joints, which leads to inflammation. If left in that condition chronically, they will cause permanent damage to their joints and may have gone past any hopes of a natural procedure or treatment for restoration and are headed to surgery of some sort.

So there is much that can be said about our diet (the foods we eat) and the link to our health and quality of life. When people make their food selections compatible with their blood type, they can reverse many of their painful joint conditions by simply losing weight (body fat). As I stated, this will ease the pressure on the joints, preventing further irritation to the joint and surrounding tissue and will ultimately reduce their pain level because of the reduction of inflammation.

Another interesting benefit from losing excess body fat or weight when eating foods compatible with your blood type is a reduction of toxicity found within the adipose tissue or fat cells. An abundance of toxins stored in the adipose tissue causes the body to stay inflamed and impede the natural healing process. So just by virtue of making food selections compatible with one's blood type, the body naturally sheds excess fat, and in the process the body goes through a natural cleansing and detoxifying of stored-up toxins.

Notwithstanding, losing weight automatically releases pressure on the knee, hips, and lower back joints, reduces pain in the joints, plus there is detoxification of cellular toxicity from the fat cells. There are even more benefits regarding pain when we eat food compatible with our blood type.

Some people may not be overweight and yet suffer from excruciating joint pain. Most everyone has residual pain from accidents or falls that may have happened earlier in their life; over time the effects of micro-tears and scar tissue buildup on the joints and surrounding soft tissue can diminish the quality of life as we age.

RENEWING YOUR MIND

- Make an honest attempt to eat foods compatible with your blood type.

- Because you are genetically unique, it makes sense to eat foods that work best for your chemistry.

- Avoiding foods that are incompatible with your blood type causes your body to detoxify and cleanse naturally.

- Weight loss is not "dieting it off," rather eating only what is biochemically available for your blood type.

CHAPTER 14

REAL PEOPLE, FANTASTIC RESULTS

"You are an inspiration in transition!" —DR. JOE

At my office in Deland, Florida, my staff informed me of a particular female client who was in extreme pain for years. She was at her wits' end and scared to death that she was bound for a wheelchair because of her painful condition. She shared that she had read my book, *Blood Types, Body Types, and You,* and wanted to submit her story about the major change she experienced in one month after making food selections for her blood type. The following is her extraordinary story; I believe it serves as an inspiration and hope to all who are in pain.

It is with much gratitude that I share my life-changing story with you.

The summer of 2009, I was shopping for a gift in a book store. As I walked through the store, a book seemed to jump off the shelf into my hands—*Blood Types, Body Types, and You* by Joseph Christiano, ND, CNC. As I was leafing through the book, I was wondering why we didn't hear more about this. While waiting in line to purchase the book, I actually sold it to the lady behind me and had to go back to get another one for me.

Once I got home, I noticed the Avoid Foods list and thought at that time that it would be difficult to follow as I didn't want to give up the foods that I liked so much, not realizing that these foods were sending my body into chaos. I have the rarest of types, AB; only 4% of people in the US have it. In the fall of 2010, my doctor sent me to a neurologist, because the pain in my body was so debilitating that something had to be done.

I had a serious lower back injury in 1962, and I was diagnosed with osteoarthritis in 1986 with the MRI tests reflecting this between every vertebra in my spine. The fall of 2010 was so difficult that two prescriptions from the neurologist and four Motrin did not cover the pain, as I was working my craft shows as an artist, and in my daily life, in general. My pain had reached the point that I was no longer able to get in and out of the bathtub and knew that if something didn't change I was headed for a wheelchair and a nursing home. The pain was in my left hip, thigh, calf, and top of my foot.

Here is where things got exciting! In January 2011, I decided to get the book out and get serious about it. *Within one month* by avoiding the Avoid Foods, *I was off all meds* and a major turning point had occurred. For months, I waited for that pain to return. I couldn't believe *the pain was gone and has not returned since*!! There was such a contrast from seriously feeling bad to feeling great that I thought, how could this have happened so fast? But after following the book and learning to *enjoy* the Beneficial and Neutral Foods, my body began healing itself.

For years I had been seeing a chiropractor for misalignment of the spine with my left hip always off to the left visually. That is over. My spine is straight. Other areas that I noticed had improved after eating for my blood type was having had an incontinence problem for a few years, I realized recently that eating according to my blood type has also affected the muscle tone in my entire body. What a relief this has been. My skin feels better and I also realized that I was no longer using eye drops due to dry eyes. To this day, I am in awe of the energy that has resulted from following this change in the foods that are for my blood type. I even sleep better and feel more rested. Having turned 70 on February 23, 2013, people don't believe it. Many people say I look like I am in my 50s. This book and the way I eat now is definitely a God-given miracle.

Of the 125 foods recommended to avoid, I was eating 51 of them. I started gradually and have avoided these foods most of the time. I have learned to enjoy the beneficial and neutral foods even more.

The better that I feel, the more passionate I have become in sharing this rewarding experience with anyone who shows an interest. It has been an incredible ride!!

My wish is that everyone could experience their healing and feel better like I have. I *highly* recommend getting this book and following it right away. I only wish I had followed it when I first bought the book instead of waiting for my condition to get worse.

Thank you Dr. Joe for changing my life and helping me be *pain-free!*

B.J. Bruner
Michigan

As I read her story, it thrilled my heart to hear how she beat the odds she was facing, just by making dietary changes to food selections aligning with her chemistry, blood type. Today she is enjoying a healthier, more energetic, pain-free life. Not a bad tradeoff for just eating—foods for her blood type that is!

YOUR BLOOD TYPE AND DIET

Most people think about blood transfusions, a hospital emergency room, giving birth, and even serious car accidents when they think about their blood type. The interesting phenomenon is many areas of your health and state of well-being is associated with your blood type. A few years ago I co-authored a book titled *The Answer is in Your Blood-type*. We listed several health problems like diabetes, cardiovascular diseases, arthritic-like conditions, and cancer, and showed how these and other health conditions are linked to a person's blood type. With a certain blood type, a person may be more susceptible to various health issues earlier in life, while another blood type may have a strong immune system, and another blood type a friendly immune system.

I see it all the time, whether among family members with varying blood types or just people in general, one individual will respond to a meal and have high energy and feel great, and a person with another blood type who ate the same meal feels sluggish and somewhat hypo-glycemic afterward. In my own family (in-laws), there is a combination of blood type O and blood type A. The blood type A family members always have some sort of cold or congestion; whereas the O blood type family member suffers rarely from this condition. Or how about the cousin or friend who can drop weight like it was ice melting in the hot summer sun, yet other family members seem to wrestle with weight control their whole lives and find it almost impossible to lose weight unless they starve themselves. And then there are people like Barbara above who learned that there is life beyond chronic pain just by making food selections according to blood type. Weight control and pain-free living is connected to your blood type and diet (the foods you select).

RENEWING YOUR MIND

- You have been amazingly and uniquely designed!

- Your blood type is the blueprint for eating foods that heal and restore health.

- You are as unique as your fingerprints, the iris of your eyes, and your blood type!

- As you strive to get healthy, remember, you are an inspiration in transition.

- Apply the knowledge of your blood type and diet and enjoy life!

- The sooner you start making food selections for your blood type, the sooner your health will improve!

CHAPTER 15

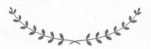

YOUR GENETIC CODE AND YOUR HEALTH

"It has been said, "You are what you eat!" I say, "Eat what you are!" —DR. JOE

The fascinating connection between your blood type and diet is the fact that it is genetic-based, not generic-based. It is superior to the one-size-fits-all concept. The way your body responds to food is based on the chemical action that takes place at the cellular level, or surface of red blood cells. This once theory-based diet plan now evidence-based is established by your genetics.

All generic-based diet plans are "old school." The genetic-based diet can easily be proven many ways, but one simple way is to feed four different people, each one with a different blood type (A, O, B, and AB) the same meal and observe them a couple hours later. One will have tons of energy and feel revitalized while another will be somewhat sleepy, a bit hypoglycemic, and another will have a little gurgling party going on in their tummy. There is no way a blood type O person will respond the same way as a blood type A or AB person eating the same food, or the blood type B individual responding to the same foods that work well for the A blood type. Different chemical response = different genetic codes. Each blood type has their own unique genetic characteristics, making them uniquely different, as do their fingerprints and the iris of their eyes.

By making food selections for your blood type, in a very short amount of time you can reduce dangerous cholesterol levels, lower elevated blood pressure, slow down the aging process, reduce body fat percentage, and boost your energy, vitality, and longevity. In addition, people can experience a reduction of inflammation in their knees, wrists, shoulders, hips, fingers, and back joints and can establish and maintain a balanced pH or cellular homeostasis (I'll talk about that later in the book) that prevents their body from becoming too acidic. Because this approach to eating is genetic-based, it naturally becomes a customized and accurate approach of eating for each individual due to the chemical responses in a person's red blood cells. What a simple answer to living beyond your chronic pain!

This advantage you have by factoring in your genetic code when it comes to what you eat and the outcome of your painful condition and overall health is by far the most accurate and scientific tool for combating chronic pain, ill health, and eventually living beyond your chronic pain.

YOUR BLOOD TYPE, DIET, AND VERSATILITY

Your blood type can aide in predicting certain diseases or conditions and serve as a great preventative measure to offset disease and illness. In our mortality study of over 5,200 individuals based on age, gender type, blood type, and diseases, we found that certain blood types had the propensity of having certain diseases earlier in life such as heart or cardiovascular disease (blood type A and AB), whereas another blood type (blood type O and B) seem not to experience such events until much later in life. We also saw the unique profiles of each blood type and how dietary changes can eliminate or greatly reduce certain illness predispositions.

BLOOD TYPE PROFILES

A Blood Type, Individual[1]

Strengths:

- Adapts well to dietary and environmental changes

Weaknesses:

- Thick blood
- Shortest life span
- Affected by stress more than other blood groups
- Sensitive digestive tract
- Vulnerable immune system
- Must avoid almost all animal protein

Health risks:

- Heart disease
- Cancer
- High blood pressure and hypertension
- Enlarged heart muscle
- Decreased immune function
- Anemia
- Liver disorders
- Gallbladder disorders
- Diabetes

Nutritional profile: abbreviated list

Beneficial/Neutral: Soybeans, tofu, and green tea have antioxidant qualities; grouper, cod, salmon, soy cheese, soy milk, lentils, broccoli, carrots, romaine lettuce, spinach, blueberries, blackberries, cranberries, prunes, raisins.

Avoid: animal fat, meat, pork, dairy products, meat-and-potato diet; kidney, lima and navy beans; durum wheat, eggplant, peppers, tomatoes, cantaloupe, honeydew melons.

B Blood Type, Individual[2]

Strengths:

- Naturally strong immune system
- Acquires most essential vitamins, minerals, and amino acids from food more easily than A or AB blood types
- Lives longer than A and AB blood types
- Second most muscular (to the O blood type)

Weaknesses:

- Some chronic medical problems such as skin disorders or foot problems

Health risks:

- Polio
- Lupus
- Lou Gehrig's disease
- Multiple sclerosis

Nutritional profile: abbreviated list

Beneficial/Neutral: meat in moderation; dairy foods; lamb, venison, cod, grouper; farmer, feta, and mozzarella cheese; kidney, lima, navy, and soybeans; broccoli, cabbage, collard and mustard greens; pineapple, plums.

Avoid: chicken, American cheese, ice cream, wheat, white and yellow corn, pumpkin, tofu, persimmons, rhubarb, pork.

AB Blood Type, Individual[3]

Strengths:

- Only blood type with two dominant traits
- Friendliest immune system

Weaknesses:

- Pattern of hormonal imbalance
- Tendency to chemical imbalance disorders

Health risks:

- Cancer
- Heart disease
- Anemia
- Autoimmune disease
- Women tend to have menstrual problems, migraines and other headaches

Nutritional profile: abbreviated list

Beneficial/Neutral: Limited to small amounts of animal protein: turkey, cod; mahi-mahi; navy, pinto, and soybeans; oat and rice flours; collard, dandelion, and mustard greens; figs, grapes, plums.

Avoid: chicken, duck, pork, venison; clams, crab, haddock, lobster, shrimp; kidney and lima beans, white and yellow corn, peppers, guava, mangoes, oranges.

O Blood Type, Individual[4]

Strengths:

- Thinnest blood
- Strongest stomach acid
- Strong immune system
- Longest life span
- Metabolizes food well
- Neutralizes cholesterol
- Low blood clot risk

Weaknesses:

- Thin blood may not clot well in brain.
- Intolerant of new dietary and environmental conditions

- Has the greatest threshold for abuse of smoking, alcohol

Health Risks:

- Strokes
- Blood disorders like hemophilia and leukemia
- Arthritis and/or inflammatory diseases
- Ulcers
- Allergies

Nutritional profile: abbreviated list

Beneficial/Neutral: Animal protein as the primary source of protein; foods rich in vitamin K, beef, salmon, mozzarella cheese, pinto beans, artichoke, broccoli, greens, figs, plums.

Avoid: pork, wheat, corn, lentils, navy beans, cabbage, Brussels sprouts, white potatoes, melons, oranges.

For a complete list of all foods, meals, snacks, and desserts, etc. for your blood type, see: *Blood Types, Body Types and You* by Dr. Christiano in the Resources Section in the back of the book.

RENEWING YOUR MIND

- It's imperative to know your blood type (see Resources).
- Your blood characteristics are blessings to know so you can make adjustments in your food selections immediately.
- Eating foods compatible with your blood type is a genetic-based approach to proper eating.
- Knowing your blood type takes the guesswork out of knowing whether you are eating the right foods to improve your health.
- Try this Acid Test—avoid incompatible foods the best you can for your blood type for 21 days, then eat those particular foods again. Notice how you feel. I promise you are going to feel horrible and at that point you can decide how many days you want to feel horrible or feel healthy. Let the evidence from the way your body responds be the proof of being on the right track.

CHAPTER 16

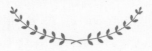

YOUR GENETIC ID BADGE

*"Your genetic individuality sets you apart
from all the rest!"* —DR. JOE

All blood types have antigens or chemical markers. These radar-type chemical markers help your body determine if a food is compatible or incompatible with your blood type. These chemical markers function as an ID badge. At the surface of each blood cell are antigens with their own chemical identification made of chains of sugar types; each blood type has its own unique code. When you ingest a food that is not compatible with your blood type, the dietary lection (protein molecule) found in the food will attach itself or glue itself to the surface of the red blood cell, and wherever it occurs in your body is where a breakdown of functionality will take place. It is through a phenomenon called agglutination (or gluing) that causes a breakdown in the functionality of any bodily system. This breakdown or dysfunction can happen in joints, stomach, intestines, liver, blood lipids—throughout your body. And of course these occurrences are usually the root causes to most diseases, illnesses, inflammation, arthritic-like pain, etc. So you can see the importance of knowing what blood type you are and making food-type selections that are most compatible.

THE ABO BLOOD TYPE SYSTEM

The 4 blood types are known as A, B, AB and O. The symbol O indicating the absence on the surface of the red blood cells of any blood group substances. The symbol A indicates the presence of a substance A on the cells, the B the presence of a substance B and the AB the presence of both substances. These substances are regarded as 'antigens' or chemical markers, analogous to characteristic antigens present on the surface of bacteria.

An antibody is named after the antigen with which it combines, preceded by the prefix 'anti-' the serum of a blood (type) group A person contains the antibody anti-B, that of the group B person contain anti-A. The serum of a group O person contains both anti-A and anti-B and that of a group AB person, neither.

To summarize the above, let's view the chart below as it illustrates the point that antigens generate antibodies.

THE ABO BLOOD GROUPS: ANTIGENS AND ANTIBODIES		
Blood Group	Blood Group Substances (antigens in Red Cells)	Antibodies present in Plasma (or serum)
O	NONE	Anti-A, Anti-B
A	A	Anti-B
B	B	Anti-A
AB	A and B	NONE

BLOOD TYPE CHARACTERISTICS

Certain blood types, like O, lack the ability to break down carbohydrates efficiently and consequently end up easily gaining excess weight and find it difficult to lose weight; whereas the A blood type has the capacity to break down carbohydrates very efficiently. And then there is the concern for cholesterol. We all have a built-in anti-cholesterol bomb or enzyme referred to as Intestinal Alkaline Phosphatase (IAP) enzyme. The secretion level of the IAP enzyme determines the affect it has on destroying long-chain fatty molecules in the blood. Blood type O has a naturally high secretion level followed by B, but A and AB have low secretion levels and are genetically predisposed to premature heart disease and cardiovascular illnesses. This is why it is most imperative to know which food types are best for your genetic individuality or blood type, so you can reverse your current health conditions or prevent them from happening.

One more example of the role your blood type and diet play is when you consider how your body responds to stress. Blood type O has a difficult time recovering from stress, as it takes longer to remove the adrenaline hormone from the blood. This is common as the O has an overproduction of adrenaline due to its "fight or flight" reaction to stress. (This is when the deep breathing technique comes in handy.) On the other hand, the blood type A individual stores more cortisol (the stress hormone) and is capable of releasing more of it when necessary when under a stressful condition allowing for a quicker recovery from stress. To prevent or reverse poor health conditions, your body must receive the most biochemically or usable nutrients it can get from a diet for it to function at its optimal level and capacity. Making food selections for your blood type will do just that.

RENEWING YOUR MIND

- Avoiding foods for your blood type will lessen or eliminate your painful condition.

- Weight loss is a by-product when you eat for your blood type.

- Put into action the knowledge you have learned!

- Making food selections for your blood type makes all the difference in a healthier you!

- The beneficial foods for your blood type are foods for healing your body.

STEP 3

LIFE IS IN YOUR CELLS

CHAPTER 17

FOOD TYPES AND pH

"Gout, arthritis, stones, heartburn, etc.—Be Gone!" —DR. JOE

I want to reiterate that *healthy lifestyle choices are your greatest defense* against illness, disease, and chronic pain, as well as for reversing current health problems. The 8 Simple Steps I have listed are vital preventative measures for maintaining good health and establishing a healthy environment.

Please keep in mind that when your body is full of poisons from medications, food preservatives, GMO by-products, pesticides and dangerous chemicals in the soil, heavy metals, junk estrogens (petroleum by-products), parasites, and other foreign toxins, it is incapable of being healed. So if you think you can take a pill and spend a day at the spa and that's all you need for your body to heal itself, you might want to think again. Your body must be cleansed and detoxified and free of health-damaging debris and toxins before healing can begin.

Because we all have to eat every day, much of the outcome of our health is determined by what we eat. As I mentioned in Step 2, making food selections that are compatible for your blood type is extremely accurate and individualized and genetically based. But in addition to blood type nutrition (diet) are foods that work in concert with the body's chemistry for maintaining a healthy pH level and thereby avoiding the dangerous and even fatal effects of acidosis or being overly acidic.

By making food selections that are compatible for your blood type and including various food types for maintaining a balanced pH balance, you can correct painful conditions such as fibromyalgia, acidosis (acidic pH), arthritis, gout, bone spurs, bunions, etc. There are certain food types that contribute to inducing arthritic-like responses and conditions in your body, and certain food types that reduce arthritic-like conditions. What goes on at the foundation of your physiology determines the outcome of your health. It is the phenomenon that takes place at the cellular level that is linked to the food types you select and the outcome of your health.

The pH, or potential for hydrogen, measures the alkalinity or acidity of a solution and is an all-important point of reference in measuring your current health as well as the determination of your future health. It is a viable standard by which potential future health risks can be measured. Your pH values are measured on a logarithmic scale from 0.00 (acid) to 14.00 (alkaline) with 7.00 being the midpoint, which is neither acidic nor alkaline but neutral.

Whether an illness or disease is acute or chronic, your body's pH level must be factored into the equation. A cellular environment that leans to being acidic in your tissues and cells is the perfect environment for developing a baseline for the disease to begin and destruction of your health to follow. Most people are not aware of this condition developing until the body starts sending out warnings—symptoms.

There are two categories of foods when it comes to blood type: Beneficial/Neutral and Avoid. One of the major benefits from making food selections for your blood type is establishing a balanced pH in the cells and tissues of your body. In addition, by eliminating foods from your diet that are in the Avoid category (these work against your blood type), you can reverse an unhealthy pH level (poor health) and then maintain a healthy pH level. In my professional opinion, making food selections that are compatible with your blood type is the most accurate way to have your food types work in concert with your body's chemistry, both from a biochemically and bio-available perspective. In other words, when you line up the foods you eat with your blood type, you are naturally feeding your body with food types that can easily and effectively be digested, assimilated, utilized, and eliminated.

Later I will provide you with a list of foods that leave an acid ash on your body's tissue as well as foods that leave an alkaline ash on your tissues. When we ingest foods that are compatible with our blood type, including alkaline-type foods, the body has a greater likelihood of overcoming painful conditions, inflammation of arteries and joints, goiter, gout, gallstones, and many other inflammatory illnesses.

The human body has a built-in natural survival mechanism for defending itself from changes in pH levels. For instance, should the body become overly acidic (and most do), the body goes into its natural survival mode and creates alkaline buffers to neutralize acid buildup or low pH level. These alkaline buffers come about from diet, the food types a person chooses. So here is the importance of what you eat having a direct correlation to the outcome of your health and condition. And of course in this instance, alkaline foods are necessary for the body to produce alkaline buffers to stabilize its pH, bring it back into homeostasis or balance. Also, there are food types that do the opposite and create an acidic baseline that forms the ideal environment for pain, disease, and cancers to develop.

Homeostasis is a condition of physiological balance where healthy, functioning cells work synergistically with the bodily systems and organs to operate smoothly. The body will do whatever it takes, even cause harm to your physical health, in an attempt to establish homeostasis. It is a natural built-in survival mechanism that comes with being a human, so you must do all you can to keep your cells in balance, or homeostasis, or there will be consequences to pay.

RENEWING YOUR MIND

- Foods for your blood type help you reach optimal pH in the tissues.

- Blood type nutrition (diet) enhances alkaline mineral reserves in your body.

- Alkaline mineral reserves protect your body's pH.

- To neutralize your pH: consume citric acid foods (lemons and/or limes), malic acid found in apples and apple cider, and even take a teaspoon or two of vinegar.

- When too acidic, eat foods like spinach, eggs, brown rice, pumpkin seeds, and fish.

CHAPTER 18

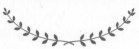

PEOPLE ARE
UNIVERSALLY THE SAME

"Try everything natural before opting for surgery!" —Dr. Joe

Sure each of us have our own uniqueness: blood type; body type; metabolic type; hair, eyes, and skin color. But take away the body's largest organ, the skin, and it's evident we all share a complex and multiplicity of cells communicating with each other 24/7. This incredible network of cells with intra- and extra-cellular functions is what we share in common. Yes, we have our own DNA, but our primary baseline for existence is found in our cells—we are universally the same.

If one of your goals in life is to live a healthy, pain-free, and long life, then you will have to learn how to keep your cells healthy, because healthy cells beget a healthy body. They work hand in hand. The best way to ensure your body of having healthy cells is to create a bicarbonate (alkaline) buffer system. And what you eat is going to make the difference in having a reserve or buffer system composed of sodium, calcium, potassium and magnesium, or alkaline minerals. When your diet lacks correct foods for maintaining these alkaline buffer reserves, your body will naturally go into survival mode when it foresees a current condition developing into a dangerous condition. Without you even being aware of this phenomenon taking place, your body taps into these buffer reserves every time your body becomes acidic or develops a state of acidosis. It is a natural way for the cellular fluids, known as extra cellular and intracellular fluid, to maintain an alkaline/acid balance. The flip side occurs should the body become void of alkaline reserves, at which time it triggers the body to send warnings or symptoms. Not being prepared, you can find your health in big trouble.

The body always seeks homeostasis no matter what harm it causes itself in the process, especially when it becomes overly acidic. Here's a common example: say your body's pH is overly acidic (well below 7.0). It naturally sends up warnings or symptoms that something is wrong. In this case you start experiencing bouts of pain, gallbladder stones, or explosive or chronic diarrhea. If left unaddressed, your body will create the perfect environment for cancers to develop. Here's a real-life story of a client of mine to exemplify the sophistication of your body's ability to protect itself when its pH becomes overly acidic.

Painful Gallbladder/Stones

I had been coaching a male client, long distance via the telephone, who was interested in dropping weight, but more so wanted to be healthier as he was approaching the 60-year-old mark. As we discussed his medical history and illness background, he mentioned that he had his gallbladder removed. I asked him what symptoms or warnings prompted his decision. He said he started having extreme pain near his stomach but it wasn't his stomach. He also said he was passing blood when he urinated. If you have ever passed blood when urinating, you know how shocking that can be. Of course the typical response is fear driven, so he called the doctor and went in for an examination. His doctor recommended a cholecystectomy or surgical removal of his gallbladder.

Remember my motto, *"Try everything else first before having surgery."* Also keep in mind that our bodies come complete—there are no spare parts. Allow me to show you how easy it is to save your gallbladder from being surgically removed and all the related digestive problems that lie ahead if you do.

Here's what takes place within your body as far as your pH is concerned and the direct relationship with a painful gallbladder. When your body's pH is balanced or in homeostasis, the proper relationship between the bile salts in the gallbladder cholesterol is in liquid form; but when the pH changes and becomes mostly acidic, the relationship becomes dysfunctional and the liquid form of cholesterol changes. This unique relationship can become dysfunctional when the gallbladder removes sodium from the bile (alkaline salts) causing the liquid form of cholesterol to become solidified and form stones. The immediate question my client should have asked his doctor was, "What can I do to keep my gallbladder?" In fact, if my client knew what to do, he would not have become another victim of whatever the doctor suggested.

Because our body was created to never make mistakes, why would the body take the sodium from the bile, causing stones to develop along with all the associated pain and discomfort? Remember that I told you how the body naturally protects itself when there is a problem. Well his body had become overly acidic and developed into a state of acidosis primarily due to his diet. Once his pH level dropped, his body switched to its natural survival mode for protection. It did so by seeking those alkaline buffer reserves. In this case, the sodium from the bile salts was needed elsewhere in the body to create an alkaline buffer to neutralize the acid buildup in his body and help restore a balanced pH. Contrary to common sense and good health, our body automatically switches to its natural survival mode, which causes the person to experience some severe bouts of discomfort and pain, the very symptoms my client was experiencing. Unfortunately, when one experiences acute or chronic pain, it generally sends that individual running straight to the doctor. Once under the doctor's care and supervision, the approach is surgery—exactly what was told to my client.

His surgery stopped the pain but did nothing about the root cause. The underlying problem was he was still overly acidic. The painful gallbladder itself was the symptom not the problem. The surgery was not necessary. The problem was my client's pH was too acidic, something his doctor never took into consideration or discussed. Are you getting the picture? If you or someone you know has had their gall-bladder removed, they will tell you all their pain disappeared and they feel great again. But the problem with that conclusion is twofold: one, the pain and stones were only symptoms of something greater going on; and two, the pH level is still imbalanced and in a state of acidosis. Surgery did not resolve the problem, it only relieved the symptoms the body was sending out with hopes of being rescued.

Let me quickly review the predicament my client is in now and the future. First of all, he gave up a body part that did not have to go. He needs his gallbladder for continuity in his digestive system, the alka-linity factors, and to make matters worse, his body is still in a state of acidosis. Does his body stop trying to protect itself now that the gallblad-der is gone—absolutely not! Because he is still acidic, his body remains in its survival mode; and with his sodium reserves gone, it starts to pull from the next available mineral to create the alkaline buffer to neutralize the acid and balance his pH—calcium. And guess where the calcium comes from, you got it—his joints and bones! See the correlation with the body's pH, bone loss, arthritic-like pain, and joint pain?

Now his body is in the process of leeching calcium from his bones. And if he doesn't correct the imbalance in his pH level, his bones will begin to decalcify; and if this happens too long, he will be dealing with another interrelated health issue—osteoporosis.

You can be proactive or reactive! The choice is up to you. If you make healthy lifestyle choices a permanent part of your life and eat foods compatible with your blood type to maintain alkaline reserves, you can prevent painful conditions like my client had and other health-related problems from developing in the first place.

To prevent the onset of painful joints, inflammation that won't settle down, diseases and illnesses, and to expect restoration of good health, you have to protect those cells. This is why it is said that we live or die at the cellular level. The wisdom here is to take care of your cells!

GALLBLADDER AND LIVER DETOX

To help your gallbladder and liver survive toxicity from medication, drugs, heavy metals, incorrect foods, refined flours, and refined sugars, etc. I have provided a simple do-it-at-home gallbladder and liver detoxification and cleansing program:

Day 1

- 12 noon: Eliminate fat from your meals after 12 noon.
- 6 PM: Drink 1 tablespoon of Epsom Salts in 6-8 oz. of water.
- 8 PM: Drink 1 tablespoon of Epsom salts in 6-8 oz. of water.
- 10 PM: Drink ½ cup olive oil with 6 oz. of citrus juice (sleep after this).

Day 2

- Upon wakening: Drink 1 tablespoon of Epson salts with 6-8 oz. of water
- 2 hours later: Drink 1 tablespoon of Epsom salts with water.

Note: Do this 1 or 2 times per year! If intense pain continues, go to the emergency room!

RENEWING YOUR MIND

- Try everything else before opting for surgery!
- Eat foods for your blood type to help balance and optimize your pH and alkaline mineral buffers.
- Balancing your pH helps reduce inflammatory joints and bone conditions.
- To balance your body's pH, try Sodium Bicarbonate (Baking Soda).
- Try Magnesium Chloride, and/or ConcenTrace (See Resources pg. 339).
- You have only one body, take good care of it!

CHAPTER 19

ACID VERSUS ALKALINE
FOOD TYPES

"You don't have to be a health nut to be healthy!" —Dr. Joe

Good health is a result of the pH balance in cellular acidity and alkalinity. As I mentioned, most people become overly acidic which over time will absolutely ruin their health. So the first questions are: what causes your body to become too acidic, and how can you neutralize or alkalize your cells?

Here I will focus on food types and their direct link to your body being either overly acidic or alkaline or balanced. But for the record, there are several other factors that contribute to being overly acidic including: stress, negative thoughts, physical work, exercise, and of course the food types you eat, particularly protein. From a holistic approach, it is the culminations of all of these factors that play havoc with your health, which can be summed up in two words—your lifestyle.

It seems quite ironic that the very things that make up the average life of every individual can be the very things that contribute to poor health such as exercise, physical work, stress or stressful conditions (chronic pain), negative thoughts, plus the type of food consumed can be the culprits that are destroying health and happiness. To make this fact somewhat easier to digest, our bodies can be overly acidic or develop acidosis when some or all of these elements are out of balance.

For example, athletes who run marathon distances or body builders who put in hours upon hours of extreme exercising in the gym or construction workers who work a lot of overtime can easily develop acidosis. How about the stressful careers and occupations of professional men and women or the stress placed upon the body and mind of a chronic pain patient who suffers day in and day out with writhing pain? Their lifestyles contribute to becoming overly acidic. When it comes to negative thoughts, it is more about when a person is *controlled* by their negative thoughts not just an occasional negative thought. Negative thinking becomes a pattern of behavior, which is actually physically destructive, especially at the cellular level, in addition to being socially destructive.

The purpose here is to learn how to balance your lifestyle, so to minimize the potentiality of becoming overly acidic and avoid premature damage to your body and health. So let's go back to food types and their link to your body's pH.

FOOD TYPES AND THE LINK TO THE BODY'S PH

Certain food types leave an acid residue or ash that contributes to a buildup of acid in your body's tissues, while other food types leave an alkaline ash or residue that neutralizes acid buildup.

It's fascinating to me how lifestyle practices such as eating and exercising can come against a person's health when, in fact, they are part of what I refer to as healthy lifestyle practices. With a closer look you can see it is not healthy lifestyle practices but a lifestyle that is not in proper balance that causes premature illnesses, diseases, and damage to health. Making food-type selections is an important aspect of our lifestyle that will improve our health and quality of life.

Let's look at the difference between acid ash-producing foods and alkaline ash-producing foods. Foods that leave acid residue or ash leave minerals that must be neutralized before the body can eliminate them. Acid-producing foods that are high in phosphorous and sulfur cause an acidifying effect. These are common foods type such as dairy products, grains, and meats. Your body can handle these acidifying minerals in moderation only. Certain fruits and vegetables that are alkaline ash-producing leave alkalizing minerals the body uses to neutralize the excess acid buildup. So one category of food types work on your behalf, while another category of food types will destroy your health when eaten in abundance.

When you consume more acid-producing food types than alkaline-producing food types for too long, high amounts of acidic residue or ash will accumulate on the body's tissue. This is an example of what happens if you go on a high protein/low carbohydrate diet. Your goal may be to lose body fat, but in the process, your body can become very acidic, which will spurn a multitude of health issues caused by a state of acidosis. Consuming a high protein and low carbohydrate diet for a short period of time will jump-start your body's ability to shed plenty of body fat, but soon the diet must return to a more balanced intake of macronutrients (protein, carbohydrates, and fats). The bottom line is if this condition (acidosis) continues too long, your body will switch on its survival mode and go straight to the alkaline reserves to neutralize the acid buildup. If the alkaline reserves are depleted, severe acidosis will develop.

The good news is, you can prevent this from happening and even reverse the condition if you replenish the alkaline mineral reserves that come from alkaline ash-producing foods, simply by selecting foods for your blood type!

RENEWING YOUR MIND

- Maintaining a balanced pH shows your body is in homeostasis or balance.

- Alkaline minerals counteract acidity in the tissue and cells.

- Make certain that you are eating for your blood type especially if you want to lose weight. This approach to eating is biochemical-friendly to you (blood type) and will not cause you to develop overly acidic tissues.

- Exercise moderately to regain the body's pH level.

CHAPTER 20

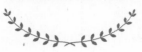

ALKALINE ASH-PRODUCING FOODS

"Feed your body what it needs—at least
80% of the time!" —DR. JOE

When it comes to making food selections for a balanced pH level, it is ideal to reach a 75/25 ratio. Whether you choose to apply this ratio per meal or snack or on a weekly basis, 75 percent of your food selections should come from the alkaline ash-producing food category, and the remaining 25 percent can be acid ash-producing foods. This approach will make a huge difference in stabilizing your pH levels, while at the same time help you maintain your health or reverse health issues.

Your primary goal is to avoid becoming physiologically acidic, or when your pH drops below 7.0. As your body remains in an acidic state it develops a state of acidosis and from there it is a downhill destructive path. Your body will become susceptible to most infections and diseases and it will be difficult to ease arthritic pain and conditions.

This category of food types contain natural alkaline minerals—potassium, calcium, magnesium, salt, etc., which neutralize acid in the body (tissues and cells). These alkaline minerals, when in abundance in the body, counteract disease and illness and arthritic conditions. Your diet should consist of alkaline ash-producing foods for a greater quality of health.

A daily diet high in alkaline ash-producing foods is a perfect fit if you are:

- Physically active
- Eating a high protein diet
- Under constant stress
- Dealing with negative emotions
- Been diagnosed with being pre-cancerous or have cancer
- Desire maintaining a proper pH balance
- Planning on being alive and well for many years

We believe it can take a minimum of three months to restore an individual's health to normal operation. To begin the healing process, your body needs: to go through detoxification, to receive proper nourishment and dietary supplementation, and exercise.

ALKALINE ASH-PRODUCING FOOD CATEGORY

Along with the following food-type categories, you will notice each fruit and vegetable shows its compatibility per blood type. I strongly suggest adding these to your diet in generous amounts daily when wanting to reverse an unhealthy condition such as acidosis or pre-cancerous and cancerous states. To individualize and make your dietary approach to healing your body most effective and to easily manage a healthy pH level, make your food selections for your blood type. Shortly, I will show you how to monitor your pH so you can determine where your physiology is at the present time and how to manage it for the rest of your life.

The goal of the following lists is to make your food selections as accurate as possible.

Fruits: almonds (All), apples (All), apricots (All), bananas (B and O), blackberries (A, B and AB), cherries (All), dried dates and figs (All), grapefruit (All), grapes (All), limes (All), peaches (All), pears (All), pineapple (All), raisins (All), raspberries (All), strawberries (All), tangerines (B and AB), lemons (All), and watermelon (A and AB).

Note: Oranges are not compatible for any blood type. *Avoid*—bananas (A and AB), blackberries (O), tangerines (O and A), watermelon (O and B).

Vegetables: avocados (All), dried beans (All), beets greens (All), beets (All), broccoli (All), Brussels sprouts (A, B and AB), cabbage (A, B and AB), carrots (All), cauliflower (A, B and AB), celery (All), chard leaves (All), cucumbers (All), parsnips (All), green beans (All), green peas (All), lima beans (O and B), goat's milk (A, B and AB), millet (All), molasses (All), mushrooms (All), muskmelon (All), onions (All), sweet potatoes (O, B and AB), white potatoes (B and AB), radishes (A and O), rutabagas green (All), green soybeans (A, O and AB), raw spinach (A, O and AB), tomatoes (O and AB), and watercress (All).

Note: *Avoid*—Brussels sprouts (O), cabbage (O), cauliflower (O), lima beans (A and AB), goat's milk (O), sweet potatoes (A), white potatoes (O), radishes (B and AB), green soybeans (B), tomatoes (A and B).

Acid Ash-Producing Food Category

Along with the following food-type categories, you will notice their compatibility per blood type. These food types should be eaten more sparingly to avoid being overly acidic, to prevent the onset of premature diseases and conditions that can lead to unnecessary surgeries, and to reverse an overly acidic state. The combination of both alkaline ash-producing foods and acid ash-producing foods with the emphasis on alkaline ash-producing foods will play a huge role in managing your pH.

Meat/Seafood: beef (O, B and AB), chicken (A, O), codfish (All), corned beef (O, B), haddock (A, B and O), lamb (All), pike (All), turkey (All), salmon (O and A), sardines (All), sausage and veal (O and B).

Note: Avoid—beef (A), chicken (B, AB), corned beef (A, AB), haddock (AB), salmon (B, AB), sausage and veal (A, AB).

Dairy: butter (O and B), cheese (All), and eggs (All).

Note: Avoid—butter (A, AB).

Grains: barley (A and O), wheat bran (B and AB), oat bran (A, B and AB), white bread (B and AB), whole-wheat bread (AB), white flour (B and AB), whole-wheat flour (AB), oatmeal (All) dried peas (All), brown rice (All), white rice (All), wheat germ (AB).

Note: Avoid—barley (B, AB), wheat bran (A, O), oat bran (O), white bread (A, O), whole-wheat bread (O, A, B), white flour (A, O), whole-wheat flour (A, O, B), wheat germ (A, B, O).

Fruits: Blueberries (All), cranberries (All), plums (All), currant (All), prunes (All), and honey (All).

Nuts: Peanuts (A, AB), peanut butter (A and AB), and walnuts (All).

Note: Avoid—peanuts and peanut butter (O, B).

Vegetables, Legumes: carob (All), corn (A), lentils (A, B and AB), squash winter (All), and sunflower seeds (A and O).

Note: Avoid—corn (O, B, AB), lentils (O), sunflower seeds (B, AB).

Note: Pork, shrimp, lobster and mammals without fins and scales should be avoided by all blood types.

To stay on top of your health, level of pain, and overall state of wellness, make certain you make food selections that are compatible with your blood type. Be certain to add alkaline ash-producing foods with your foods that are compatible to your blood type when seeking a balanced pH. Acid ash-producing foods can be eaten in moderation but eliminated if you are highly acidic or are in a state of acidosis. Once reversed to an alkaline-acidic balance, you can add the acidic ash-producing food to your diet.

*Learn how you can plant your own blood type vegetable garden with non-GMO, non-Hybrid and Heirloom vegetable seeds specific to your blood type. (See: Home-Grown Blood Type Vegetable Garden Package in the Resources section in the back of the book or go to: www.bloodtypegardens.com.)

TEST YOUR PH

Determining your urine pH indicates how well your body is responding to the foods you ate the day before. If you eat acid ash-producing foods, your urine pH reading the next morning should be somewhere around 5.8-5.5. This acid reading shows the most favorable physiological response to acid ash foods and indicates that you have alkaline mineral reserves available. Should this reading change over time by becoming alkaline (over 7.0 pH), it may indicate that your alkaline mineral reserves in your body are very low and need to be replenished.[1] You can do this by drinking ionized water (alkaline water), eating more alkaline ash-producing foods, by adding an alkaline mineral supplement, or both.

You can test your body's pH yourself. You first need to purchase pH paper test strips from your local pharmacy. A popular brand is pHydrion Papers. The paper that registers between 5.5 and 8.0 is most suitable. You want to check for fluctuations in your urine pH readings day to day. You can test yourself as often as you want, but testing over a 2-week period is most effective.

THREE-DAY MONITORING

Day One

1. Begin monitoring urine pH with the first void in the morning after you have eaten foods you usually eat. The numbers you get for Day One will serve as a baseline.

2. Eat only acid ash-producing foods (meats, grains, nuts, and so on). You may need to plan ahead for these meals if you ordinarily eat generous amounts of vegetables.

3. Drink only water if possible. If not, then limit coffee, tea, cola, or other beverages to 2 cups or less each day. Avoid alcoholic drinks and fruit juices.[2]

Day Two

1. Repeat Day One. Retest in the morning. Eat only acid ash-producing foods. Limit water and other beverages.[3]

Day Three

1. Retest in the morning. Resume your regular food selections after you take a reading on Day Two's food.[4]

PH SCALE OF ACID REACTION (IN THE BODY)								
Acid								**Alkaline**
Total	Very	Moderate	Slight	NEUTRAL	Slight	Moderate	Very	Total
0	1-2	3-4	5-6	7	8-9	10-11	12-13	14

To perform the pH balancing act, keeping your alkaline versus acidity in check, you will need to add alkaline ash-producing foods to your daily diet, which then moves you away from the high protein, no or low carbohydrate diet. Now you have a better opportunity of being healthy while losing weight for the long haul.

The food-type lists in this chapter are plentiful enough to help you with your decision-making process for customizing your meals and snacks to fit your specific needs, improving your health, strengthening your cells, ridding your body of toxins, and preventing the onset of unforeseen illnesses and diseases. To custom design your own meals and/or snacks, simply pick and choose which food types and groups you prefer.

Having a better understanding of the blood type diet and how it is so very individualized, plus the knowledge of your pH and the importance of maintaining a pH balance—life just got better for you.

RENEWING YOUR MIND

- An acidic environment is dangerous and damaging to your health.

- Acidosis is an overly high acidic condition that can lead to painful conditions, inflammation, and ultimately cancer.

- Achieve an alkaline acidic balance for maximum health and pain-free living.

- Make it a practice to test your pH so you can prevent the premature onset of disease and illness.

- Hydrate with alkaline water when possible.

STEP 4

COLON CLEANSING

CHAPTER 21

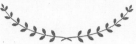

COLON HEALTH

"The 'dirty inside story' you were never told!" —Dr. Joe

BATHROOM MATTERS

Colon health is probably the least talked about topic, leaving most people uninformed and therefore in grave danger of premature diseases, illnesses and worse—death! According to 2013 health statistics, more than 140,000 new cases of colon and rectal cancers were diagnosed in the United States, making it the third most common form of cancer among Americans.[1]

Because our colon has everything to do with the outcome of our current and future health, it behooves us to know what to do to keep it functioning well. There are two simple things we must do: stop polluting and clean up the existing pollution. If you do not take care of your colon, there is no doubt that you will face unnecessary health-related illnesses and have a less-than-acceptable quality of life, even to the point of premature death.

Sounds rather serious, doesn't it? Well, it certainly is! Just think about all the many medications you have been taking over the months and years for treating symptoms like pain and inflammation. People on a regime of medications are actually polluting their bodies, in addition to all the environmental toxins, junk estrogens from petroleum products, toxic metals, and incompatible foods for your blood type. The question is, "How much pollution or toxicity does it take before our body stops functioning naturally and can no longer heal itself?"

Once you realize the crucial role your colon plays in enhancing your health or destroying it, you will be motivated to stop polluting it and instead clean it up.

So let's take a trip through the digestive system and see how it works.

THE PATH OF A MOUTHFUL OF FOOD

Elimination is one of the most important yet probably the least understood bodily function. That's probably because it's not something we talk about. In fact, it's a taboo subject—one, we avoid. Who wants to talk about fecal matter, waste, bowels, and parasites? We'd rather talk about beautiful, healthy, and pleasant things. But as you'll discover, the elimination process, when functioning properly, leads to beauty and health. And when functioning improperly, it can lead to lack of energy at best, pain and discomfort, sickness and disease at worst. So it's worth putting aside the taboos and talking about it, don't you think?

When you swallow a mouthful of food, it goes to your stomach to be converted to a semiliquid form called chyme. After the food (chyme) leaves your stomach, it travels through the small intestine. The chyme passes from the small intestine into the colon through the ileocecal valve. The colon, a large muscular organ five feet long, is located at the end of your digestive tract.

||||||||||||||||||||||||||| HEALTHY TIP |||||||||||||||||||||||||||||

The colon has three basic functions:

1. To absorb water and electrolytes from the chyme
2. To move waste material out of the body
3. To store the waste until it is evacuated

Imagine your colon being like a curvy roller coaster. The passengers (chyme—consisting of food, water, liver excretions, and the like) enter the roller coaster car, which starts at the bottom (the cecum). The colon begins to move the car up the ascending colon with involuntary wave-like contractions, a process called peristalsis.

Billions of friendly bacteria in our colon break down some of the materials we can't digest, and from this process come nutrients like vitamin K and a few of the B vitamins. This bacterial team also breaks down some of the protein into less complex substances.

When the car reaches the hepatic flexure at the top of the ascending colon, it does a 90-degree turn and goes across the transverse colon, still climbing to a higher level. From there the car does another 90-degree turn at the splenic flexure and heads straight down the descending colon to the end of the ride at the sigmoid colon and the rectum.[2]

During the digestive process, the chyme is moved through the colon by the peristaltic muscular action in the colon walls. In this process some positive bacteria and moisture are withdrawn.

HEALTHY TIP

In the past several years many health authorities have agreed that most illnesses are linked directly to either a blockage in the colon or poor bowel function. Well-known bowel specialist V. E. Irons claims, "In my opinion there is only one real disease, and that disease is autointoxication—the body poisoning itself. It's the filth in our system that kills us. So, I'm convinced that unless you clean out your colon you will never regain vibrant health."[3]

Dr. Norman Walker states, "Good health not only regenerates and builds the cells and tissues which constitute your physical body, but also is involved in the processes by which the waste matter, the undigested food, is eliminated from your body to prevent corruption in the form of fermentation and putrefaction. This corruption, if retained and allowed to accumulate in the body, prevents any possibility of attaining any degree of vibrant health."[4]

Dr. Walker concludes by saying, "Not to cleanse the colon is like having the entire garbage collection staff in your city go on strike for days on end. The accumulation of garbage in the streets creates putrid, odoriferous, unhealthy gases which are dispersed into the atmosphere."[5]

The matter that begins its downward journey through the descending colon is called feces. Toxicity and waste from your blood as well as putrefying bacteria are carried in the fecal matter to the sigmoid colon, the rectum, and then out of the body.

If the colon is healthy and operating normally, it will eliminate the toxic waste materials easily and regularly, without strain. But if your colon is not in good operating condition, it will not eliminate properly. This causes those toxins in the feces to build up in your system and begin damaging and destroying your health.

THE COLON AND YOUR HEALTH

Just like mixing flour and water to make a paste, a similar paste-like substance can build up in your colon. If the food selections you make are not compatible to your blood type, if they are processed and not fresh and full of roughage, or if they are from a dairy-source, they are difficult for your colon to move through the digestive tract. Consequently, slime builds up on the porous walls of the colon, which actually plasters the walls like paste.

As the buildup continues over the years, your body can no longer absorb the nutrients and nutritional supplements through those walls. Often, because of the buildup on the inner walls, there is barely enough space for food and fecal material to pass through. Believe it or not, most people are walking around malnourished—even those who eat regularly and take their vitamins. They lack energy because their colons are clogged. According to Dr. Norman Walker, a specialist in colon health, "The consequent result is a starvation of which we are not conscious, but which causes old age and senility to race toward us with the throttle wide open."[6]

"In the fifty years I've spent helping people to overcome disability and disease, it has become crystal clear that poor bowel management lies at the root of most people's health problems. In treating over 300,000 patients, it is the bowel that invariably has to be cared for first before effective healing can take place," says Dr. Bernard Jensen.[7]

HEALTHY TIP

Several unnecessary illnesses are common today because of the conditions of our colons. Hopefully, recognizing them will raise your level of awareness and motivate you to clean your environment and avoid the dismal consequences.[8]

- Constipation—caused primarily by insufficient dietary fiber
- Diverticulosis—a pouch-like sack or ballooning in the intestines, caused by increased internal pressure and weakening of the bowel wall
- Diverticulitis—inflamed diverticula
- Colitis—inflammation of the colon, also known as irritable bowel or spastic colon, when the inner lining of the colon becomes inflamed
- Hemorrhoids—dilated veins in the anus and rectum
- Stricture—Chronic narrowing of the colon passage due to inflammation
- Prolapsed colon—falling of the transverse colon because of accumulated waste material and general deterioration of colon health as a result of poor colon hygiene

Frighteningly, your internal digestive, absorption, and elimination system can be turned into a garbage dump that will pollute your body and weaken and destroy your health.

When the fecal matter cannot move regularly through the colon and be disposed of, they ferment and putrefy just as if a sewage system were backed up.

Think of the environmental health problems that would exist if the sewer system in your city was backed up and ignored by the sanitation department. It wouldn't take too many days before the sewer system became a cesspool, polluting the entire environment and causing parasitic infestation and disease. Your city would become extremely toxic—not an acceptable environment in which to live.

Well, the very same results occur when your digestive system is not kept operating properly. Many people are in a constant state of fatigue, lethargy, and sickness because of their neglected interior sanitation system.

AUTOINTOXICATION

If your colon is congested and has been plastered for a long time, it probably is not functioning normally. In fact, it cannot function normally! Your body cannot rid itself of the rotting fecal matter because it's impacted onto the walls, and that slows down your body's ability to eliminate efficiently. Ultimately your congested colon is actually poisoning you and producing toxicity throughout your entire body.

This condition of your colon also affects your body's ability to absorb nutrients properly. In fact, the small amount it is absorbing is toxic because a congested colon is polluted and very toxic. Your entire digestive system becomes a toxic dump, and these toxins are carried via the bloodstream to other areas of your body, introducing you to another entire host of health problems.

According to Dr. Bernard Jensen, autointoxication is "the result of faulty bowel functioning which produces undesirable consequences in the body and is the root cause of many of today's illnesses and diseases."[9]

The colon seems to be able to endure this infectious and toxic condition without much pain because it lacks nerve endings. Unfortunately, many of these abnormalities are allowed to develop because they go unnoticed.

Harvey W. Kellog, MD, says, "Of the 22,000 operations I personally performed, I never found a single normal colon, and of the 100,000 performed under my jurisdiction not over 6 percent were normal."[10]

According to Dr. Walker, "If a person has eaten processed, fried, and overcooked foods, devitalized starches, sugar and excessive amounts of salt, his colon cannot possibly be efficient, even if he should have a bowel movement two to three times a day."[11]

There's another interesting perspective to understand: the correlation between a healthy, functioning colon and lower back pain. I know that when our patients and clients do a thorough colon cleanse they somehow have less or no back pain. From his book *Prescriptions from Paradise*, Dr. Carlos M. Viana, OMD, CCD, writes, "In fact, I have never treated a person with lower back pain, especially one with a supposedly herniated disc at L4/L5, who did not also suffer from constipation."[12]

RENEWING YOUR MIND

- Drink enough water for your body weight—stay hydrated.

- Foods compatible with your blood type will assist in proper elimination.

- Constipation is detrimental to the health of your colon.

- A normally functioning colon will prevent autointoxication.

CHAPTER 22

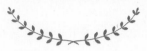

PARASITIC INFESTATION

"Be careful who you have over for dinner!" —DR. JOE

Approximately 300 types of parasites thrive in the intestinal tracts of people in America today.[1] It is quite possible that you are walking around, a human buffet for tiny little invaders that did not receive your VIP invitation.

June Wiles, PhD, parasite expert, stated, "Parasites are vermin that steal your food, drink your blood, and leave their excrement in your body to be reabsorbed into the bloodstream as nourishment."[2]

Whether a microscopic single-cell parasite or a four-inch worm, these little parasites love to eat whatever the host is eating—but they are first in line. After they are thoroughly fed, we get what is left over, mainly in the form of the parasite's excrement.

Parasites can become your unwelcome guests through shaking hands and playing with your pets. They can be transferred by adults, children, and food handlers. You can get parasites by eating uncooked meats and raw fruits and veggies.

HEALTHY TIP

Parasites come in all types—pinworms, tapeworms, hookworms, roundworms, ringworms, and giardia lamblia, a tiny microscopic parasite being studied by scientists today in America. "One out of every four in the world is infected by roundworms, which cause fever, cough, and intestinal problems. One quarter of the world's people have hookworms, which can cause anemia and abdominal pain. A third of a billion people suffer from the abdominal pain and diarrhea caused by whipworms."[3]

Parasites are easily passed around by millions of people each day just by coming in contact with one another. And if you consider the millions of people who eat at restaurants every day, you can see how parasitic contact can become overwhelming. Usually if one member of your family has them, then everyone will get them.

Among children in temperate climates the pinworm is the most common parasite. Overcrowded schools and daycare centers aid in passing these parasites to others. These conditions have caused an increase in pinworm infestation in children. One child in six having pinworms used to be the norm, but now this infestation is up to an astounding 90 percent of children in America.[4]

While there are more than 300 varieties of parasites, only about 25 varieties can be seen without a microscope. Those that can be seen without a microscope include pinworms, hookworms, roundworms, and tapeworms. These critters build colonies in the rectum and colon and cause them to be irritated and raw.[5]

In the Southern states, the hookworm is most common. This uninvited body destroyer causes abdominal pain, diarrhea, malnutrition, apathy, anemia, and even undevelopment in children.

The problem of parasites is much more widespread than health professionals ever dreamed it could be. Centers for Disease Control experts point out that doctors are at a loss when it comes to the diseases brought on by parasites, because their training and schooling is very limited on parasitic infestations.[6] Doctors are reluctant to admit to the microbial epidemics like parasites and clogged colons. Most people are ignorant of the health problems that can be caused by parasites.

It is a medically known fact that impacted, clogged intestines and junk-filled and sugar-filled colons are the two major causes for the epidemic breakout of parasites. This condition makes a perfect place for all worms of all sizes to thrive. Intestinal parasites and worms can cause you to be sick. For instance, if you are housing giardia lamblia, you may end up doubled over with abdominal pain or vomiting, belching, fever, and exploding diarrhea. Unfortunately, antibiotics do not affect the giardia.

Many parasites do not penetrate the intestinal wall, but they leave your bloodstream full of their excrement. If they cannot enter your intestinal region, they can still dump toxins in your body and can challenge your immune system.

TRANSIT TIME

Transit time is the amount of time it should take for a healthy colon to transport the nutrients into the body for nourishment and then dispose of the toxic waste that remains. The volume of food and liquids ingested as well as the condition of the colon determines transit time. In a healthy colon, the transit time should be no more than 16 to 24 hours. Elimination should occur once after each full meal. If the body takes longer than the normal transit time to eliminate the waste, then toxic buildup begins.

Once toxic buildup occurs, your digestive tract becomes a real breeding ground for parasites. These little guys are looking for a home to raise their families—and they love to multiply and produce lots of kids.

The faster the roller coaster ride, the less time the parasites have to multiply. The average incubation period for a parasite is 36 hours, so if your roller coaster car is traveling at the prescribed 16 to 24 hours, then you are in good shape. On the other hand, if your colon's transit time is that of the average American, then you have serious problems, as the average is 96 hours![7]

Dr. Tom Spies, recipient of the American Medical Association's (AMA) Distinguished Service Award, reminds us, "All the chemicals used in the body—except for the oxygen we breathe and the water we drink—are taken through food."[8] Our food selections have a direct link to the way the bowel responds. Studies have shown that the regular intake of refined carbohydrates or sugars and the lack of most Americans to include sufficient fiber in their diet slows down the transit time, increases the buildup of waste and fecal matter, and promotes putrefactive bacteria.

Through neglect or being unaware, thousands of people suffer painful bouts from diverticulitis, irritable bowel syndrome, celiac sprue disease, cancer of the colon, and many other chronic diseases because of the poor sanitation service they are giving their bodies. An unhealthy colon impacted with sugars, burgers, fries, and white-flour products is at the root of these poor-health problems.

Many medical experts consider it a myth that a plaque-coated colon or parasitic infestation could be directly linked to illness, disease, and sickness. This attitude may be due to the fact that there is no patented medicine or drug for quick relief of an impacted colon. In fact, medicines can't unclog an impacted intestinal tract or colon.

You might want to consider that your colon and intestinal tract may be totally coated with plaque, add in some parasite, and there is good reason for feeling lousy, weak, and unhealthy. So do you have foul breath, feel achy, or have sore joints or regular headaches? Then there is a good chance your colon needs some cleansing.

Perhaps by this point you are screaming, "What can I do?"

RENEWING YOUR MIND

- Get enough fiber—30 mg. daily.
- Drink pure water only.
- Eat foods compatible with your blood type.
- Get regular, moderate exercise.
- Reduce as much stress as possible in your life.

CHAPTER 23

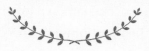

COLON CLEANSING

*"Spring and Fall colon cleansing will revitalize
your body, inside and out!"* —DR. JOE

There is no doubt in my mind that colon cleansing and detoxifying is vitally important to attaining good health and preventing premature illnesses and diseases. Colon health is the bedrock and foundation to a healthy life.

After researching the many herbal laxatives and cleanses, I formulated my own colon cleansing system, INNER OUT which my wife and I have done twice a year for more than 15 years. (See: INNER OUT in the Resource section in the back of the book.) Instead of taking some capsules for 20 to 30 days that give mild diarrhea or soft stool, a thorough colon cleansing system is what is most needed.

To give you an idea of the powerful and efficacious results that my colon cleansing system provides, I want to share with you a letter from a mom who tells about her son who was miraculously cleansed after months and months of medications and antibiotics being administered to him after having half his scalp replaced because of an auto accident.

I just reordered mine a couple of days ago. I have personally been using this product (INNER OUT colon cleansing system) since 2002! I saw Dr. Joseph Christiano on TV talking about feeling sluggish, skin problems, indigestion, etc. and the body's need for a colon cleanse. He named a lot of reasons why we all need to cleanse, but he mentioned the necessity of cleansing if one has been on a lot of medication/antibiotics.

Well, my 25-year-old son had been in a car wreck, went in a coma, had half of his skull removed and put in the freezer. For 3 months he was given several strong medications. When they put his skull back on, he was given intravenously the strongest antibiotics available and multiple kinds so his body wouldn't reject his skull. Now this is the reason I became so sold on this unique colon cleanse that actually scrubs your colon walls.

You see, almost two years after my son's wreck, his complexion was so bad. It was hard for him to accept because he never had acne as a teen and was always complimented on his beautiful face. After watching the show I decided to place an order for myself and my son. I did mine first and honestly felt 20 years younger! Then my son, Joshua, did it. I was thinking about all the prescriptions he had been on for so long, but had completely forgot about the feeding tube he had for 9 months. The day his feeding tube was placed, they ran a bag of some turquoise radioactive dye through his system to ensure that it was placed correctly.

I was in absolute shock and awe as the colon cleanse scrubbed all 9 feet of his colon. For three days he produced 9 feet of turquoise, you know what! *Immediately* I remembered that radioactive dye hanging from the pole next to his bed. I also remembered that at the nursing home when they would disconnect a feeding bag from his tube that it would drip on the floor. If it would dry without being wiped up, then it would take a razor blade, not a paring knife to remove it. It was like hard rubber when it dried. Joshua's colon was lined with this stuff for 2 years!

This amazing product scrubbed it clean, like new. His complexion immediately cleared up and even better than that is his memory became so clear, no more short-term memory block. He was back to normal and we became completely sold on this God-breathed product of Dr. Joseph Christiano's, and I have many friends and family using it now.

Thank you, Dr. Christiano!

Debra H.

I was so humbled to read this letter of the health benefits both the mom and her son experienced from my INNER OUT colon cleansing system. As you pursue a healthier pain-free life, I hope you will consider colon cleansing.

For information about my INNER OUT colon cleansing system, go to the Resources section in the back of the book.

ELIMINATE WHITE FLOUR AND REFINED SUGAR

People cannot easily digest the white flour that breads, bagels, rolls, pastas, and even pretzels are made of. Though these foods are common, they are not good for your body. White flour in any product is dead flour, and it provides empty, useless calories. Let me show you what I mean.

Wheat in its natural form in the fields is full of nutrients for human consumption. It lacks nothing and does not need to be fortified. White flour fell into the hands of the food manufacturers. In the process of getting that beautiful white flour into your mixing bowls and then onto the dinner table, all fiber is stripped from it. During its journey to the supermarket, a bleaching process is necessary, which destroys the nutrients. In obvious acknowledgment that good things have been removed, manufacturers then add some synthetic nutrients and call it "fortified, enriched" flour. Many innocent shoppers assume that everything on the grocery shelves is good for them. But that's not true.

White flour is a major contributor to weight problems, low blood sugar, and a congested colon. The body treats white flour as sugar; when it is eaten too often and too much, the body experiences an over-insulin response, which contributes to slowing down its metabolism (the very thing you need running at high speed for weight management). Consequently, white flour causes us to get fat.

Besides working against our metabolism, our bodies are not getting the nutrients or fiber content that were originally in the wheat when it was in the garden. Over time the body breaks down because it hasn't been receiving the nutrients it requires. Last but certainly not least, this "wonder food" has clogged the colon and allowed it to become the human hotel for all the parasites in town.

Perhaps you thought junk foods were limited to candies, cakes, and chocolates. Well, white flour and white-flour products must be included in this category. Do yourself and your family a favor, do not buy any more white-flour products. Instead try eating rice flour bread, even Ezekiel bread (sprouted grains and wheat), buckwheat, barley flour, spelt, millet, or 100 percent rye bread. If you eat wheat bread, keep it to a minimum. But if you are a blood type O or B, avoid it completely. If you love pasta, try spelt, rice flour, and Jerusalem artichoke pasta as alternatives.

ELIMINATE REFINED SUGAR

Refined sugar is basic table sugar and is found in candies, pastries, cookies, pies, sodas, sweetened iced tea, doughnuts, ice cream—the list goes on and on. Many processed foods contain a high amount of sugar. Refined sugar is not digestible; it contributes to tooth decay, obesity, depression, hyperactivity, hypoglycemia, weakness, cancers, and much more. Does this sound like something you would recommend to someone you love—even yourself?

|||||||||||||||||||||||||||||||| **HEALTHY TIP** ||||||||||||||||||||||||||||||||

Many of the clients I have counseled seemed to be hooked on soda. I had a client who used to drink 10 to 20 12-ounce cans of soda a day. By the way, that is about 450 cans per month. With 12 tablespoons of table sugar in each can, that equates to 180 tablespoons of sugar per day, or 5,400 tablespoons a month.[1] That is just like adding a slew of chemicals and some water to a 10-pound bag of sugar and drinking it every month. Can you imagine the damaging affect all the acid had on her pH level and association with chronic pain? Could that be the link to her headaches or difficulty losing weight? You better believe it—that and more!

NATURAL DETOXIFICATION—EATING FOR YOUR BLOOD TYPE

Eating foods that are compatible with your blood type allows your body to go through a detoxification period because of the blood type association with the wall of the digestive track. You will experience tremendous relief in the digestive tract, relief from intestinal pain and discomfort, and you will be able to assimilate your food more efficiently. Consequently, you will have little to no gastrointestinal problems. You will have a greater sense of being satisfied after eating because of the improved digestion and absorption abilities. There will also be fewer opportunities for parasitic infestation to take hold—all that comes just by making food selections that are compatible to your blood type.

The information regarding this area of your health might seem somewhat gross at first, but ignoring the condition of your colon will not change the sobering importance of it. The body that you were given to live in is a very precise piece of machinery that requires constant attention. Your body is so incredibly intertwined that it is impossible to ever assume that each gland, system, and organ will somehow take care of itself. When one area breaks down, the others are affected. With all the advantages of technological advancements, new medical discoveries, procedures and remedies, plus advancements in dietary and nutritional research and alternative medicine, we should strive to be as healthy as we can.

I am not suggesting that your marvelously designed body is in need of some external concoction or methodology to improve its own natural and innate ability to survive a lifetime. But the damage that you cause to your body by the use of medications for pain and other conditions or turning the other way and thinking that someday it will improve on its own is formidable. That kind of thinking is responsible for keeping your physical body in an unhealthy condition and robbing you of a life that can be enjoyed to its fullest.

The quality of your life is solely dependent on the highest level of optimum bodily function and performance. When the colon is neglected, overlooked, or abused, there is absolutely no hope for any life that resembles what you were created to enjoy. So start today, keeping your colon in tip-top shape!

RENEWING YOUR MIND

- Make food selections compatible for your blood type to assure the most accurate nutritional baseline.

- Do a thorough colon cleanse twice yearly.

- Consider hydrotherapy.

- Take magnesium citrate supplements to aid the peristaltic action of the colon for proper transportation of waste and food through the colon.

- Maintain regular exercise to aid proper colon function.

STEP 5

A STRONG IMMUNE SYSTEM

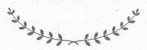

THE IMMUNE SYSTEM: ARMED FORCES AGAINST INVADERS

"As the military protects its borders, your immune system protects you!" —DR. JOE

When I was an early teen, my brother Bob and I played the board game Risk with our friends. From the onset of the game, players are surrounded by invading armies out to overtake them. We used our armies to attack the territories of others and to protect our territories from attack. The key to protecting our own territory from invaders was building up our armies so they outnumbered the enemy. And so it is in the real world. Ever since you took your first breath, your body has been attacked by various invaders trying to get inside your body. These invaders are turned away by your army, the immune system. Without that army, your body would be extremely vulnerable to sickness, disease, and crippling pain.

Every human body is equipped with an amazing capacity to protect and preserve itself. Those of us who are in pursuit of a life of vitality and good health must tend to our immune system. It is our own health protector and is necessary to support a strong, healthy, disease- and pain-free body.

UNDER ATTACK!

Encased within your body's largest organ, your skin, is a massive collection of 60-plus trillion cells. These cells are different from each other and are uniquely arranged to form the varying organs and systems, which, when all working together in harmony, allow your body to function properly. So keeping happy, healthy cells is imperative for pain-free living.

For us to survive, let alone live healthier lives, our cells must be nourished, cared for, and maintained to function properly in their biochemical realm. The cells must also be protected from the continual attacks of their enemies. Picture your body as the universal ballroom where those 60 trillion cells get together and dance perfectly, and you will see why they are so adamant about not allowing any uninvited guests to their functions.

The problem is, your body, like the players in Risk, lives in an extremely hostile and unforgiving environment. From your first day on this planet, your body has been surrounded by vicious enemies continually trying to find ways to enter to harass and disturb your party. You must be able to recognize these enemies in order to resist their attempt to crash your body's "Health Party" and avoid the diseases they bring with them. These enemies include yeast and fungi, which attempt to establish colonies, reproduce, and eventually cause your body to decompose. Also on the uninvited guest list are viruses that afflict your body with illness and disease. And of course, this list would not be complete without bacteria, which putrefy and spread death. As you can see, we are walking around in enemy territory.

If you think these enemy attacks are the only means by which health can be ruined, you are wrong. Cancer, for instance, occurs when our cells reproduce themselves uncontrollably. The polluted air we breathe, the polluted water we drink, and the processed foods containing preservatives and additives we eat also damage our cells and weaken our immune system. We cannot escape this endless warfare of invaders battling against our immune systems.

Many times my profession calls for me to travel. Just by boarding an airplane I can come into contact with global germs, not to mention the physical contact I may have with people from around the world, possibly exposing me to a large number of viruses, fungi, and bacteria. Have you attended a formal event or public event where someone shook your hand right after sneezing in their own? It might have been healthier to salute that person instead!

The very fact that we are alive is proof that our immune systems are actively working on our behalf. So this area of your makeup must be shored up and fortified. With such a variety of enemy forces marching against our borders, it is absolutely necessary to build up a strong defensive army to protect our own cells and then to identify, seek out, and destroy all intruders.

Have you ever wondered why some of your family members seem to catch everything that comes along, while others do not? Why does your grandmother, who suffers with heart problems, and the old man up the street with emphysema, and the toddlers in the daycare class you teach seem to be the first ones to catch the flu and other viruses going around? Why does the body try to reject the transplanted organ that could give it new life? Or why do kids get chicken pox and other childhood diseases only once? The answers can be found by studying our immune system.

HOW THE IMMUNE SYSTEM OPERATES

"Seek and destroy" is a military offensive strategy routinely used by the infantry. And that is exactly what your immune system does in response to an attack. At the first sign of an invader, such as bacteria, the immune system sounds the alarm, which alerts the defense system to seek and destroy the enemy.

The immune system has a tremendously sophisticated method of determining whether a substance is foreign or friendly. Not only is it able to recognize millions of enemy molecules attempting an attack, but it can produce molecules and cells to form a line of impenetrable defense to counterattack the enemy and drive it off.

|||||||||||||||||||||||||||HEALTHY TIP||||||||||||||||||||||||||||

The immune system is as complex in its structure as the brain and nervous system. It can distinguish the enemy from its own "invited guests." It can remember previous experiences—like a round of chicken pox—and prevent that experience from happening again. And it has at its command a sophisticated array of weapons.

|||||||||||||||||||||||||||||||||||||||||||||||||||||||||||||||||||||||||||||||||||||||||||||||||||||||||||||

Chemical markers, or antigens, are found on every cell in the body. Blood type antigens are some of the most powerful antigens in the body. The blood type antigen identifies whether the invader is a friend or foe by checking out the antigen located on the invader.

Lymphocytes are a type of white blood cell that actually patrol the circulatory system and the areas of fluid immediately surrounding the cells. They are the main functional cells of the immune system.[1] They consist mostly of T cells, responsible for cell immunity, and B cells, responsible for antibody production. T cells travel widely throughout the body. They help the body defend against foreign substances, and they surround damaged or diseased body cells.

The B cells, too, are called into battle. Specialized B cells produce antibodies, and these antibodies function like anti-aircraft missiles, firing their antibodies on invading enemy viruses and diseases. These B cell antibodies join forces with the T cells to surround the diseased cells and destroy them.

While this internal war is raging on your behalf, you might experience some soreness or even pain in your joints as well as inflammation and redness in the lymph nodes. When these symptoms occur, don't panic; it is just your body's way of reacting to biochemical casualties taking place. It's actually a wonderful indication that your system is doing its job.

THE CLEAN-UP CREW

Another group of white blood cells, macrophages, are then recruited into action. Macrophages are large immune cells that devour invading pathogens and other intruders. The direct orders for these guys are to eat everything in sight that is covered with antibodies. Then, after they eat, they explode. The circulatory system then cleans up the mess by carrying the deceased to the elimination department.

The amazing immune system always keeps an adequate supply of antibodies in reserve ready for the next attack. Some of the lymphocytes have a good memory; in case there is ever another encounter with that flu virus or other disease, the alarm will sound immediately, and victory will be sweet one more time. This is what we refer to as immunity to a disease. It is why children seldom catch the same childhood disease twice.

It's no secret how vicious the immune system can become, but at the same time it can be very sensitive. In fact, it will turn on itself and attack the body's own cells, should they become malignant. Thankfully, there are cells known as suppressor cells, which keep the body's cells from attacking its own. But if these suppressor cells are not functioning properly, the body's healthy cells can be attacked. The result is called autoimmune disease.

As you can see, the immune system is crucial because it seeks and destroys every uninvited invader that enters the body with murder on its mind. So it stands to reason that keeping our immune system in tip-top operating condition should be our number one priority.

The strength of the immune response to the invader is dependent on the strength and condition of the host's immune system. If the immune response is inadequate, the invaders will not be destroyed. Instead, they will multiply and invade the cells of the body. If your immune system should quit functioning one day, you would be left with absolutely nothing to protect your body from viruses, bacteria, and infections. That would be like playing Risk with no armies to protect your territories against invaders. As you can imagine, you would lose!

RENEWING YOUR MIND

- Maintain food selections that are compatible with your blood type.

- Don't smoke.

- Exercise regularly.

- Maintain a healthy weight.

- Control your blood pressure.

- Avoid alcohol or drink in moderation.

- Get adequate sleep.

- Practice good personal hygiene; wash your hands frequently and cook meats thoroughly.

- Get regular medical screening tests for your age group and risk category.

CHAPTER 25

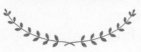

ENEMY INFILTRATORS

*"Uninvited guests will ruin your house
party every time!"* —Dr. Joe

As powerful and yet versatile as the immune system is, like any army, it is also susceptible to infiltrators that undermine its power and try to bring about its collapse. Of course, viruses and bacteria try to get in, but other infiltrators are more covert. If we can pinpoint these infiltrators, major or minor, we can work on eliminating them from our lives.

OUR POLLUTED ENVIRONMENT

Accompanying our turbo lifestyles are the continual challenges that war against our immune system from the outside—the air we breathe, the water we drink, and the food we eat. The population growth in America has also caused a real health problem—overcrowded highways with thousands of trucks, cars, and buses sending toxic fumes into the atmosphere and polluting the air we breathe. That's not to mention the smokestacks from the industrial plants spewing into the air millions of chemicals just ready to be inhaled.

Our cells are bombarded with toxins that are weakening our immune systems, causing respiratory infections, breathing problems, and a host of other ailments. Our drinking water, with all its chemicals, pollutants, and bacteria, is another means invaders get into our bodies.

The pollutants have free radicals, which are impaired molecules that try to attach themselves to the good cells in our systems, and over time they break down cellular function. If our cells are continually challenged like this, they will weaken and allow disease and illness to have their way. Symptoms like headaches, itching, rashes, or fatigue can be signs of the beginning stages of an immune system breakdown.

Even the foods we eat can work against our immune systems. Most people will eat anything on their plate before carefully considering potential health risks that nitrites, nitrates, food additives, processed foods saturated with chemicals, or rancid, oil-soaked fast food can have.

I am convinced that eating foods compatible to a person's blood type will save a lot of unnecessary trips to the doctor, lower healthcare costs, and help us enjoy a more desirable lifestyle. Just as we have no control over the color of our eyes, neither do we have control over which foods are better for us biochemically than others. It's in our genes.

For example, if a blood type A person consumes dairy products, there's a good chance the result will be an overabundance of mucus in the respiratory system and the lining of the airway passages. This is due to the lectins found in those particular foods that are not compatible to the A blood type antigen. The subsequent mucus buildup then creates a breeding bed for infections and bacteria. Give the same dairy products to people with blood type B, and they will not experience any such reactions because those particular foods are compatible to their blood type antigen.

It is amazing to realize and appreciate how perfectly designed the blood type antigens are and how powerfully they work in the immune system. With it being said that the immune system can defend against most attacks of any uninvited intruders, then it is just a small percent of invaders that get into our bodies that cause all the diseases and illnesses. Though only a smaller amount of invaders can enter our bodies, we should do all we can to protect our immune system. We should do all we can to fortify our immune systems.

Research is proving that there is increasing bacterial resistance to many antibiotics that once cured bacterial diseases readily. Due in part to the rise of resistance to antibiotics, the death rates for some communicable diseases (such as tuberculosis) have started to rise again.[1]

ENDLESS PHARMACEUTICALS

Unfortunately, most people run to the doctor for a prescription every time they get sick or experience some form of symptomatic reaction. Our bodies have not been designed to ingest these dangerous chemicals—nor do any of them cure. But one thing they do for certain is cause our bodies to become poisonous and toxic. This approach to healing or "getting better" needs to go!

In His masterful design for His human creature, Yahweh (God) created the human body with the precise ability to heal, detoxify, and energize itself. It is up to us to do all we can naturally to preserve our health. Conventional medicine and its approach to our health brings with it a mentality that it is easier to swallow a pill than to eradicate the root cause.

In her book *Poisonous Prescriptions*, chemist Dr. Lisa Landymore-Lim states, "Given that a poison is *any* substance that when introduced into or absorbed by the body injures health or destroys life, most of today's pharmaceutical preparations, because of their harmful effects, may be labeled poisonous."[2] Dr. Landymore-Lim provides insight into the poisoning nature of pharmaceutical drugs. And guess what the side effect of most medicines is—a challenged immune system.

Medications have other side effects as well. Just read the insert from the pharmacy when you get your next prescription. I'm astounded by the fact that many people would never dream of reading the side effects of the medications that the doctor prescribes, but they will argue tooth and nail that taking vitamin C could be detrimental to one's health.

Not only are antibiotics often unnecessary, but they frequently destroy the helpful intestinal bacteria and deplete certain vitamins. A study by doctors at Cleveland's University Hospital has shown that even aspirin compromises the infection-fighting ability of the white blood cells.[3]

People need to realize that although antibiotics may be necessary to treat certain bacterial infections, they can have detrimental effects on the body. They should be used only when absolutely necessary—not for viral infections. A doctor friend from Indianapolis confessed to me that throughout his medical training years, the primary thing he was taught was how to put bandages on the symptoms. The causes of the problems remained untreated.

I am not bashing the medical community—I believe there is a place for conventional medicine. But my prayer is that someday the conventional medical community and the alternative medicine community will join hands and work together for the betterment of the American people. I am of the mindset that it is my responsibility to do all I can from a natural perspective to prevent and maintain the health of my body. If, and only if, I have tried everything natural but have not succeeded, then I consider visiting the medical community.

Prevention, precaution, and protection preserve your health. If you are trying to keep your immune system strong and healthy so it can keep you strong and healthy, avoid unnecessary medications and work on building your immune system.

DAILY STRESS

Due to our fast-paced society, all of us are exposed to lifestyles that are saturated with stress. Our bodies are living daily under stressful conditions, but I'm sure this is not news to you. You understand the stress of family life, raising children, spousal relationships—and, of course, the relatives. Then there is the stress in our occupations—the endless pressure from deadlines, sales meetings, appointments, bosses and coworkers.

Almost everyone experiences financial stress to some degree—the cost of living, insurance rates, gasoline prices, childcare, the national economy woes. Many people have more days in the month than they have paycheck to cover expenses.

Though stress is not a bug that infiltrates our immune system, it certainly affects it. Stress can weaken our immune system and keep it from operating efficiently, making us more susceptible to attacks from viruses and bacteria. Pollution, drugs, stress—these infiltrators can weaken the immune system. Then little problems can lead to bigger problems. Serious diseases are linked to immune system failure.

AUTOIMMUNE DISEASE

While our magnificently designed immune system is responsible for protecting our body from sickness and disease, we have learned that it is continually being challenged by the pollutants in the air, water, and soil, plus all the drugs and medications we ingest.

Taking medications for too long a period of time can cause the body to build up an immunity to the medication. With sleeping pills (not barbiturates), for instance, after taking them for a while, the body requires more of them to have the same effect. After years of being challenged by different medications, the immune system can turn on its own cells. The worst case scenario is that a person may contract an autoimmune disease.

Autoimmune diseases are simply the results of the immune system breaking down. It can no longer read the radar screen properly, and consequently it cannot distinguish friend from foe. The system then makes auto-antibodies, which attack its own cells. They destroy their own organs and cause inflammatory responses. Some examples of autoimmune disease include Amyotrophic Lateral Sclerosis (Lou Gehrig's disease), Chronic Fatigue Syndrome (CFS), Rheumatoid Arthritis (RA), AIDS, and Lupus—all very painful.

CANCER

Cancer is the "C" word, as many refer to it with fear in their eyes. What is this dreaded disease? Within each cell is a code, generally referred to as DNA that is duplicated over and over again as the cell reproduces. It is extremely important to protect this code in order for the cell to reproduce correctly. This protection is totally dependent upon the immune system. If a carcinogen, or cancer-causing agent, makes it past the immune system protectors and is allowed to disturb or distort the code and cause it to reproduce in an uncontrolled and erratic manner, then that cell becomes mutant. The result may well be the development of a malignant tumor and the beginning of cancer.

When the immune system detects the beginning of cancer, it begins its seek-and-destroy mission. The immune system works in two ways to fight cancer. If the carcinogens have not yet entered the cell, the immune system sends out the seek-and-destroy troops to stop them before they take hold. A healthy immune system will also work to destroy the mutant, cancerous cells that have already formed in the body. So if you can supercharge your immune system, it can defeat and in some cases reverse the cancer process.

The immune system is vital to the fight against cancer. With its help, the body can fight the battle against cancer—and in many instances, be victorious. Immunotherapy is a new way of treating cancer that uses our body's natural defense system, the immune system. It has been used successfully to treat several kinds of cancers, including skin and kidney cancers and some lymphomas. As more and more research is done, we will become better able to help our immune system win the battle against cancer.[4]

So, is there anything we can do to keep the immune system as healthy as possible? The good news is that we can definitely shore up our immune system and keep it working at top efficiency.

RENEWING YOUR MIND

- Make food selections for your blood type.
- Implement healthy coping skills to de-stress.
- Avoid antibiotics the best you can.
- Get regular exercise.
- Reduce medications, pollutants.
- Take dietary supplements (Immune Support, see Resources).

CHAPTER 26

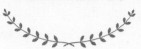

Maintain a Strong Immune System

*"To boost your immune system simply eat —food
selections for your blood type!"* —Dr. Joe

If we truly understand the life-protecting function of our immune system and the seriousness of its potential breakdown, then we cannot help but be concerned about protecting it. Millions of people suffer from frequent colds, recurring bouts of the flu, headaches, migraines, hay fever, sinus infections, and allergies—all obvious symptoms of a challenged immune system that is possibly losing its battle against the enemy invasion.

The body creates 200,000 new immune cells and thousands of antibodies every second in order to be strong enough to defend its host—you and me. This means that millions of cells have to be rebuilt every day. It is absolutely imperative for our bodies to get the adequate nutrients essential for this day-to-day combat. It would behoove everyone who reaches for medications and drugs that mask the symptoms to reconsider their damaging effect on the immune system, then take the proper steps to naturally build the immune system instead.[1] As I mentioned over and over, if you are in need of various medications for pain, inflammation, etc., make certain that you are supplementing your diet (blood type) with immune-boosting supplementation.

You can fight the battle within your body during the period of taking medication to avoid many of the horrific side effects that come with the territory.

Many things help strengthen the immune system, including exercising, minimizing medication, avoiding hazardous environmental pollutants, lessening contact with radiation (X-rays included), and learning how to de-stress. Taking antioxidants also helps to eliminate free radicals from the system. But the one aid to strengthening the immune system that I believe is the baseline or foundation in which to build upon has to do with blood type.

HEALTHY IMMUNE SYSTEM AND THE BLOOD TYPE CONNECTION

All cells have a chemical marker used by the immune system to determine whether the cell is friend or foe. These markers, referred to as antigens, are part of the cell's chemical makeup.

When various foreign bacterial, viral, and parasitic antigens enter our bodies, the immune system responds by producing antibodies to destroy the intruding enemy antigens. The B cells in the immune system produce these antibodies. When the T cells recognize the production of antibodies, they bind to the foreign antigens to help fight against these intruding antigens. The enemy antigens try to change or disguise their appearance in order to evade capture and annihilation. Of course, the immune response is so accurate that the T cells and the antibodies simply glue themselves to the enemy antigen, clumping them together for easy disposal.

But some immune systems are friendlier to a particular enemy antigen than others. The immune army of people with blood type A, for instance, sometimes has a problem identifying certain invaders that have the same A-type antigen that the immune army has. That makes it more difficult to pick up the invader on the radar screen.

The blood type A system has to work to fight off the attack of foreign antigens with A-type antigens. As the immune system works to escort out the intruder, the person may get sick and have to fight the sickness. This same process would occur when another blood type person was fighting off foreign antigens that carried the same blood type antigens.

|||||||||||||||||||||||||| HEALTHY TIP ||||||||||||||||||||||||||

The antigens that determine your blood type are the most powerful in the body. When these different blood type antigens are functioning properly, they become the immune system's greatest army. Remember, the reproduction of most of the antibodies usually requires the presence of the invaders, either through a vaccination or an infection. But this is not the case with blood type antibodies. They are produced automatically by the body and are always available to do battle. This makes them invaluable.

Each blood type responds to invaders such as bacteria, virus, or parasites in a uniquely different way. So it is important to be aware of your blood type to watch for certain immune system responses. Specific associations exist between blood types and autoimmune disorders. Because of the association that blood type has with the immune system, it is normal to find that certain diseases are more common to certain blood types.

The blood type O person is a predominant sufferer of arthritis, which is an autoimmune disease. That means the type O person must be aware of the responses that take place when eating certain foods, such as white potatoes, which can induce inflammatory reactions in the joints.

The blood type A person will often experience arthritis, but with puffiness, painfulness, and debilitating breakdown of multiple joints. The blood type A individual can experience these responses to stress as well. In fact, they are known to be more high-strung and may, therefore, innately bring on rheumatoid arthritis-like symptoms.

Multiple sclerosis and Lou Gehrig's Disease are more common to blood type Bs because of their tendency to contract slow-growing viral and neurological disorders. Some researchers believe that these two diseases are caused by a virus contracted at a young age that has B-like antigens.

Because the immune system of blood type Bs cannot produce anti-B antibodies, these viruses can slowly develop over many years. This is a classic example of how the invader has fooled the immune response.

AB blood types are at high risk for these B-like diseases as well because their bodies do not produce anti-B antibodies either.

IMMUNE SYSTEM HEALTH THROUGH A HEALTHY DIET

By now I'm sure you agree that strengthening the immune system is a good idea. There are a number of ways by which we can do this. One of the ways to strengthen the immune system may be something you have not considered before, but I consider it to be extremely important: because our cells have only what we put into our bodies to work with, the choices that we make about the foods we eat are critically important to our immune system.

Contrary to popular belief, even when we attempt to get proper nutrition by eating fresh, wholesome foods, it is impossible to receive the same abundance of nutrition from them today as people did 50 plus years ago. Many of our parents and grandparents ate foods from their gardens or from the garden of the local vegetable seller. My father and his father grew their own vegetables, so their meals were prepared with fresh produce, grown in uncontaminated soil.

Today, damage to the soils and water from chemicals, pesticides, and fertilizers has virtually left the vegetables that are sold at grocery stores throughout our country deficient in nutrient and mineral content due to the fact that the soils are deficient—far from what it was like back in the day of our parents and grandparents.

This is why I offer *non*-GMO, organic and heirloom vegetable seed packages that are compatible with a person's blood type. There is nothing like eating a fresh healthy salad with your favorite lettuce and chopped veggies or a nice steak dinner with your favorite vegetables that came from your own garden! (Visit: www.bloodtypegardens.com or call 1-800-259-2639.)

HEALTHY IMMUNE SYSTEM—DIETARY SUPPLEMENTATION

Things just aren't the same as they were, so it behooves us to take precautionary measures to safeguard our health. When we consider the fact that the average diet of people in our society consists of fast foods and processed foods, it becomes imperative that we enhance our dietary nutrition with dietary supplements. This approach is a nutrient safeguard due the nutrients lost through depleted soils, improper food preparation, poor food choices, missed meals, sickness, or stress.

|||||||||||||||||||||||||||||| **HEALTHY TIP** ||||||||||||||||||||||||||||

Keeping your body healthy is dependent on a strong immune system. The following list includes only a few of the foods, spices, and herbs that can play an important part in strengthening your immune system. The immune system of each blood type varies from the other and may have unique nutritional requirements.

Type A

- Spices/Herbs—Tamari, Echinacea
- Vegetables—Maitake mushrooms, garlic
- Legumes—Lentils
- Nuts/Seeds—Peanuts and/or nut butter

Type B

- Spices/Herbs—Kelp, rose hips
- Vegetables—Garlic, potatoes, cabbage, leafy greens, and yams

Type AB

- Spices/Herbs—Kelp, Echinacea
- Vegetables—Garlic, potatoes
- Soybeans/Legumes—Lentils

- Nuts/Seeds—Peanuts and/or nut butter
- (All compatible vegetables for types A and B are compatible for type AB except tomatoes. Type AB can enjoy them without any negative reactions.)

Type O

- Spices/Herbs—Kelp
- Vegetables—Garlic, broccoli

||||||||||||||||||||||||||||||||||||||||||||||||||||||||||||||||||||||||||||||||||||||||||||||||||||||||||||||||||||||

You are unique, and so may be your specific nutritional requirements. Some people require a specific combination of nutrients for their specific condition. Let me use the following powerful example of utilizing specific nutrients for a very painful condition called fibromyalgia.

Fibromyalgia (FMS) for the most part is considered a rheumatic-like disorder characterized by chronic achy muscular pain with no obvious physical cause. It seems to affect most commonly the lower back, neck, shoulders, back of the head, upper chest and thighs. It is often difficult to pinpoint the exact area of pain, and it can affect almost any part of the body.

The most distinctive feature of fibromyalgia is what is known as the "trigger points," 18 spots that have been identified by the ACR (American College of Rheumatology) as extremely tender to normal touch. To confirm a diagnosis of fibromyalgia, a patient must have tenderness at 11 or more of these trigger points.[2] The stiffness and pain that is usually described as throbbing or shooting, even stabbing, is greatest in the morning, but can occur throughout the day as well.

Symptoms experienced by fibromyalgia sufferers may range from chronic headaches, skin sensations and irritable bowel syndrome, to anxiety, palpitations, memory impairment, dry eyes and mouth, irritable bladder, dizziness and impaired coordination. As the condition worsens, most sufferers are unable to perform daily tasks such as ironing, lifting items or climbing stairs because of the day-to-day painfulness of their condition.

Fibromyalgia most commonly seems to be experienced by women, though men can suffer from it also. It strikes about 3.4 percent of American women and 0.5 percent of American men.[3] It appears that this condition starts in young adulthood and worsens as the individual ages. Though there is no real evidence of its cause, it seems to be related to the immune system.

The problem I have observed when working with fibromyalgia clients is that although they may have been struggling with the disorder for many years, the only treatment they have received from their doctors has been continual prescriptions for medications that never seem to relieve their suffering.

While conducting several wellness workshops for those who suffered from fibromyalgia, I heard their horror stories of being medicated by their physicians with everything from anti-inflammatory medication to antidepressants, sleeping pills, and even morphine. Nearly all of them were overweight due in part to the lack of exercise, but also because of the reactions to the variety of medications. They often had lifeless eyes and appeared drugged. In fact, they were human medicine cabinets. Most said that after they had been treated (in some cases as long as 20 years), their physicians let them go and suggested they receive psychotherapy because they were hypochondriacs. (These symptoms are similar to people with TMS.)

The following is a story of a young mother who lived in New York and had been suffering with fibromyalgia for 10 to 15 years. She was always tired and had terrible mood swings. Her condition became so bad that she had to leave her employment. Once she was diagnosed with FMS (years after she had the first symptoms), she started doing her own research to find help.

When she contacted me, I told her about a natural approach to beating FMS. I recommended that she first start with a colon-cleansing program to remove parasites, toxins from medications, and bad bacteria, and to help get her digestive system back in good operating order. I recommended an energy booster that works naturally to help balance her hormones, and suggested she drink a protein shake twice a day—one specific for her blood type. Plus, I gave her suggestions for changing her diet to foods that were compatible with her blood type. I also recommended aloe vera juice for stimulating her immune system.

She was very faithful to do the things recommended and experienced improvement within the first two to three months. A little over one year later, she contacted me and said, "I keep waiting for everything you suggested to stop working, but I keep getting better and better. I have more energy, much less pain, and really enjoy my life again. I can't remember ever having a day where I could say I felt good. Now I have strings of days when I feel great!" She is happier and healthier than she has been for years.

I am in no way suggesting that you should not see your physician or that supplements should be taken in place of medical treatment. But as for me and my perspective—*try everything natural first!*

My advice is to first consider the natural alternatives available to you especially if you are suffering from continued pain and energy loss. If after exhausting all you can naturally, then see a conventional medicine physician. When taking preventative measures to be healthy, the trips to the doctor's office will be cut back significantly. It is worth the time, energy, and money to try everything natural first because you are investing your resources into your health not wasting them on dangerous medications that only treat symptoms. An ounce of prevention is worth a pound of cure. But maybe a pound of natural prevention is the cure!

DIETARY SUPPLEMENTS FOR COMBATING ARTHRITIC-LIKE PAIN

Some people, because of their condition or the demands on their health, might require more or less than others in both supplementation dosage and variety. I would recommend that you keep your supplementation plan as simple but as individualized as possible. Contact a naturopathic doctor or healthcare practitioner who is experienced in natural health for a consultation.

To help strengthen the immune system and the heart and to build the body to resist infections and cancer and painful conditions, supplementing your diet will greatly enhance your health. In an ideal world we would eat only those foods that are compatible for our blood type, exercise regularly, and get eight hours of sleep a night. But that might not represent your real world. So what can you do to make your world healthy for you and your family?

STAY ON THE DEFENSE

Healthy cells are imperative for keeping your immune system in tip-top operating condition. The immune system is the health protector and the major contributor to a longer and greater quality of life. There is not much hope for a healthy, vibrant, and energetic life without giving constant attention to protecting and nourishing your cells with proper nutrients, exercise, and foods that are compatible to your blood type.

As a boy I learned a great lesson from playing Risk. If I wanted to win the game, I had to learn the significance of building a strong defensive army on each of the territories I owned. In doing so, I was able to defend and protect my territories from the enemies that came to take away what was mine.

Keep your immune system strong! You will be ready to defend against those nasty health-robbing invaders and win should that ugly face of ill health pop up and try to take your health away.

RENEWING YOUR MIND

- Get adequate sleep.
- Make food selections for your blood type.
- Avoid late hours.
- Reduce stressful conditions and people.
- Exercise regularly.
- Colon cleanse to; remove bad bacteria and toxins from your body.
- Kill off parasites.

EXERCISE

CHAPTER 27

BENEFITS FROM EXERCISE

"Exercise is NOT a form of punishment!" —DR. JOE

It's impossible to hear the words "body" and "exercise" without think-ing that we could be doing something about our flabby triceps or bulging bellies. Most people think of exercise as putting their bodies through sweaty, painful movements—an almost acceptable method of physical self-abuse—just for the reward of looking better. Beauty, looks, the body beautiful! Is that the only reward for exercising, or is there more?

It has now been shown that exercise or physical activity is more of a means for preserving and protecting our health than reducing waist-lines. Medical reports, studies, and research now support the fact that many health-related benefits accompany physical activity. In fact, going back as far as 1996, the Surgeon General's Report on Physical Activity and Health says that inactivity is a serious nationwide problem.[1]

The stronger the body, the better we are able to do everyday tasks, recreational activities, and sports. The better shape our heart and lungs are in, the greater stamina we will have. Many people have difficulties performing simple tasks such as yard work or bowling because their bodies are not fit. In fact, they are unfit.

Some people have preexisting physical conditions that limit them from performing certain exercises or tasks. But even having an injured

lower back or knee or other physical limitation is not necessarily a reason to avoid exercise completely. A smart approach to exercise allows
you to enjoy the benefits from exercise even if you are limited in what
you can do.

If you have physical limitations, consult with an exercise physiologist, a personal trainer, or a health club that has competent instructors
who can work with you to come up with appropriate exercises.

Exercise is not limited to building biceps and reducing waistlines. It
is a necessary part of everyone's lifestyle to prevent osteoporosis, heart
disease, adult diabetes, and problems associated with carrying extra
weight. It is now almost impossible to separate preventing illness from
having a fit body. They are dependent on each other and are necessary
elements of regular body maintenance.

The focus for incorporating regular exercise into your lifestyle
should be twofold: 1) improving your health through prevention of illness and 2) maintaining a leaner, calorie-burning body.

As you incorporate exercise into your life, remember that not everyone can be (or wants to be) a Mr. or Miss America. Setting your sights
on a realistic goal will save you a ton of frustration and disappoint-
ment, especially if your hope is to look like the model on the cover of
Cosmopolitan or *GQ*. Let me tell you that "computerized cosmetics" have
a lot to do with the flawless photos you see. Besides that, if the model
you are trying to look like is 5 feet, 11 inches tall and you are 5 feet, 3
inches, well....

Think for a minute of an old-fashioned slide rule. We want to slide
away from the end of the scale that represents total abuse and neglect
of our bodies while at the same time avoiding the opposite extreme
of total obsession with our bodies. Our purpose is to find the happy
medium that will give us satisfaction for the immediate but also protection and preservation of our health for the future.

PHYSICAL BENEFITS—A HEALTHY BODY

Some time ago a client once asked me what I did for my own personal training. After I told her how I trained and how often, she said

in dismay, "You're going to have to keep that up the rest of your life!" I chuckled to myself because at the time I had already been training for nearly 40 years!

Exercise is not limited to attaining the body beautiful, even though that reason tops the list for most people. Exercise makes the human body healthier. As the individual participates in an exercise program, the body experiences an increase in core body heat, which in turn causes the body to eliminate toxins by sweating. Plus, exercise is the only means of flushing the lymphatic system, which means less of a chance of infection.

Exercise promotes circulation of blood throughout the entire body, delivering oxygen and nutrition to the cells and muscles, then dispelling carbon monoxide through heavy breathing. The lungs also get a thorough workout when a person exercises.

Through exercise, the musculoskeletal system is strengthened, including soft tissue-like ligaments and the tendons. The joints then get a break because stronger muscles do the work of holding the body. I'm certain if you are dealing with a bad knee or elbow or even a hip, every time you take a step or bend to move, you feel tremendous pain in that joint. As you add exercise to your daily life, you will eventually find relief from pain as the muscles and soft tissue bear most of the load instead of the joint.

As the overall physical condition of the individual improves, so does the body's resistance to injury, sickness, and disease. Exercise stimulates the immune system, thereby contributing to building the body's defense mechanism against sickness, disease, and fatigue. Regular exercise allows the body to utilize insulin properly and speeds the metabolism to burn calories more efficiently. All these contribute to a healthier body.

After you start exercising regularly, when you miss a workout or two, you will notice that your body almost craves that stimulation. Your body was not designed to be sedentary; it was designed to be physically active. Your body will adjust to the stimuli you give it and will continue to improve as you increase the stimuli.

"WHOLE PERSON" BENEFITS

Why do people choose to make exercise a consistent part of their lives? For myself as well as many other exercise keepers (those who keep exercise in their life), the answer is not only the health benefits (though they are tremendous) but the positive inner experience associated with the exercise itself. When people reach this inner mindset of enjoying the exercising itself—and many do reach that point—they become instinctive exercisers.

Certainly we all need to gain the health benefits, and the shapelier bodies that come from exercising can't hurt either. These external benefits keep our motivation up. But if we focus solely on them, we can lose the motivation that keeps us on track for the long haul. To become instinctive exercisers we must learn to enjoy the movement and the exercise itself. To appreciate the warmth in an injured or hurting joint when exercising is like none other. Learning to do so is imperative to move from sedentary living to a life of regular exercise.

|||||||||||||||||||||||||||| **HEALTHY TIP** ||||||||||||||||||||||||||||

Motivating Factors of Exercise

External benefits

- Exercise reduces the risk of disease.
- Weight management is easier with exercise.
- Exercise requires a disciplined mind.
- Exercise meets an expectation.
- Exercise brings relief to your joints.

Internal benefits

- Exercise feels good.
- Exercise brings enjoyment.
- Exercise satisfies your desire to keep fit.
- Exercise gives immediate gratification.

One way to view exercise motivation is on a continuum from external benefits to internal benefits. External motivation places emphasis on doing a behavior for its rewards or outcomes, thereby focusing on the result. Internal motivation focuses on doing a behavior for its own sake.

Setting clear-cut goals is necessary to avoid distractions and to keep focused. If you have been bored before with exercising, most likely you became bored because you never developed clear, specific goals. It is impossible to get totally absorbed in your exercising if you do not know where you are going. I have overheard people at the gym say that they were going to get on bikes and just pedal away. That often is a sign of someone who has not made clear-cut or precise goals, but is just wandering.

When I used go to the gym, I was not the most sociable person there. That's because I stayed focused on what I was doing. I'm self-taught on how to concentrate during my workouts. When I perform a particular exercise, I mentally envision the muscle functioning. I actually see it contract and relax. In this way, I enjoy the movement and the exercise itself.

Because concentration can easily be disrupted in an open gym environment, you might try using a computerized machine at a health club because it is personalized and usually in a private room. Hiring a personal trainer who understands your interests and goals can also help you avoid distractions so you can get totally absorbed in the exercise.

Keep in mind that reaching certain goals comes by focusing on the purpose not the task. For example, I would set different goals in my walking program. Some days my goal was to walk fast and other days to slow it up and enjoy the landscape. The next day I might feel social, so I ask Lori to go with me. By varying my goals, my interest stays high, and I stay motivated.

The mental connection that is involved in your fitness journey will give control to the "yes" voice. Emotionally, people climb out of the dark valley of low self-esteem and negativity. Because I've benefited and feel better, I will treat you better and encourage you. I can now be all that I can be. I like myself, so I can risk liking you.

Finally, sharing all this positive emotional and psychological good with others will enhance your well-being. You feel good, so you can be a good neighbor and a good friend. Because you have learned how to overcome the physical and mental obstacles, you can challenge and encourage yourself to tap into your hidden resources.

The first step to all these positive benefits to exercising is a new way to look at freedom.

FREEDOM TO FEEL AND BE YOUR BEST

For years I have asked my clients their definition of freedom. Though their answers varied, the common denominator was being able to do whatever they wanted to do without any restrictions.

This definition of freedom is actually a form of bondage. *Real freedom comes from having boundaries, not being without them.* Let me explain.

Suppose for a moment that your goal is to lose weight. Can you imagine eating as much as you want, whenever you want, wherever you want, without any restrictions—and expecting positive results? That would be impossible. You would find that what you thought was freedom was not. As a matter of fact, the very mindset that freedom means no boundaries has contributed to the health problems many Americans are troubled with today.

Let me show you freedom from a different perspective. I'm sure you remember your mom saying, "This medicine might not taste good, but it's good for you," or "In life, there will be times when you have to do certain things that you don't want to do." Well, she was right. And she was talking about freedom.

HEALTHY TIP

The more you exercise, the more physical and mental energy you experience. The more often you exercise, the more endurance and muscular strength you develop. Everyday activities and tasks become easier. You enjoy the changes taking place in your body. You like what you see in the mirror. Your attitude is more positive, and your perspective toward other areas of your life is broadened.

||||||||||||||||||||||||||||||||||||||||||||||||||||||||||||||||||||||||||||||||||||||||||||||||||||||||||||||||||||||||||||

Because you feel the physiological and physical improvements, you can't help but like yourself. You have disconnected the negative messages and now accept only the positive, so you have a whole new attitude that has lifted your self-esteem. You find yourself to be more assertive.

Now you can start living life again. The giftedness and talent that has been suppressed for some time begins to surface. You have stopped complaining about pain and the people around you enjoy your company because of your positive outlook on life as well as your inspirational conversations and words of encouragement.

In other words, you have been freed—you are experiencing freedom because of the boundaries you put on yourself to exercise whether you felt like it or not.

There is something to be said about the magnetism that exists in people who are physically fit. They naturally and automatically demonstrate commitment, discipline, balance, and control. They exude good health and vitality. This discipline and balance naturally flows to the other areas of their lives, bringing harmony.

You will appreciate your progress through exercise and a positive mindset for overcoming pain and discomfort. Freedom is the result you get when you are doing the things that you ought to be doing.

RENEWING YOUR MIND

- Keep your motivation with a positive attitude.
- Recognize your value and importance to others.
- Overcome negative thoughts and focus on benefits from exercise.
- Exercise to strengthen weak and painful joints.
- Exercise to fight disease and illness.

CHAPTER 28

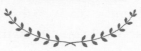

HOW TO START EXERCISING

"The quickest way to start your exercise program
is by getting off the couch!" —DR. JOE

If you are dealing with chronic pain and want to get your body stronger so it can function better, or perhaps you are interested in making it healthier for a greater quality of life, then there is no question that regular exercise pays huge rewards. Once you understand and accept that physical fitness can contribute to providing you with a better quality of life, the only thing left is to be educated in exercise technique and what works best for you.

Let's start with some basic principles to help you on your fitness journey.

PROGRESSIVE FITNESS PRINCIPLES

Principle #1: Exercise should always be based on your physical limitations! Listen to your body. Exercise a minimum of three times weekly. Anything fewer than three days per week, and you might find it difficult to lose body fat. On the other hand, you should start out slowly but progressively, especially if you dealing with joint problems, pre- or post-surgery—always allow what your fitness condition dictates. Too much too fast will cause potential injury and burnout, and will lead to dropout.

Principle #2: Exercise for a minimum of 15 minutes. We know that as few as 12 minutes of exercise per workout can produce cardiovascular improvement. When you feel you can do more, add minutes to your workout time.

Principle #3: Warm up and cool down. Ideally, a 10- to 15-minute warm up of walking or cycling prepares the heart, lungs, and muscles for a vigorous workout. It raises your core body temperature, which puts your body into a fat-burning mode. After your workout is over, it is a good idea to slow down the pace and cruise for about ten minutes or so. Stretching is a perfect way to cool down. This gives your internal machinery time to recover at an easy pace. Cool-downs also assist in eliminating much of the lactic acid buildup (soreness) in the muscle tissue incurred in the main exercise time.

Principle #4: Drink 8-10 ounces of water about 20 minutes before each workout session. Then continue to sip water during the workout. It is important to rehydrate your system immediately after exercising, to replace the lost water through sweat and evaporation. The time to hydrate yourself is not when you feel thirsty, but throughout the activity.

Pay close attention to the environment around you. If you are exercising outdoors and it's hot and humid, you might be wise to go indoors or pass on the workout completely. Your body will have a difficult time cooling itself down in those conditions. Make sure you drink enough fluids (water) throughout the day, every day.

Principle #5: Practice safety during exercise. Monitor your heart rate throughout your workout sessions and stay within your ideal range. (See Cardio Chart on the gym walls or on the machines.) Remember to breathe freely. Sometimes people subconsciously hold their breath while exercising—you won't last long in the gym or on planet Earth if you do that. Holding your breath can cause elevated blood pressure, too. Concentrate on exercise technique and form.

Principle #6: Do a variety of exercises. Follow a baseline of exercises at least three times per week, but on the other days, mix it up. Do some biking or hiking, go on walks, or play some tennis or fun activities. Keep your exercise time interesting by varying your activities.

Principle #7: Make exercise social. Include family and friends. The nice thing about exercising is that it can be social. Some prefer to go it alone, but for the majority it is fun to share this positive experience. For couples who go for evening walks, exercise is a way to share being outside while sharing from the inside with each other.

I want to add a special emphasis on the physical fitness condition of your children. They must start off as young as possible, plus they need leadership from their parents. This will cause you to get on the ball too. If you are a parent, get involved in your children's lives and do physical activities with them. Get the kids away from the TV and the video games. Take them outside and play tennis or volleyball, take walks, throw the football around, get involved in recreational activities at the local YMCA or exercise together at home. Get creative for boys or girls. Their health is in your hands.

HEALTHY TIP

Seven Fitness Principles

1. Exercise at least three times weekly.
2. Exercise at least 15 minutes.
3. Warm up and cool down.
4. Drink 8-10 ounces of water 20 minutes pre-exercise.
5. Practice safety during exercise.
6. Do a variety of exercises.
7. Include family and friends.

By the way, your program should have the simplicity and flexibility to be conducted in the privacy of your home or at a health club, if you prefer. It need not require complicated or expensive equipment. Your program should also be time savvy. Most people do not have a lot of time to spare, so keep it short but effective. Then you will be able to stay motivated for the long haul.

THREE COMPONENTS OF AN EXERCISE PROGRAM

Obviously, it is impossible for me to design a personal exercise program for everyone who reads this book, but I can give you an idea of what your body requires and what an exercise program should provide you. (Contact Dr. Joe at 1-800-259-2639 for a consultation.)

All exercise programs should consist of the following three components: aerobic conditioning; strength training, and flexibility training. Let's look more closely at each.

Aerobic Conditioning. Exercises that enhance the cardio-respiratory system—walking, jogging, cycling, and stair climbing—are aerobic conditioning. (This does not refer to aerobic high-impact classes.) Aerobic exercising is doing something that keeps your heart rate sustained at 60 to 70 percent of your maximum heart rate.

The benefits of aerobic conditioning include strengthening the heart and lungs, improving circulation, improving cholesterol ratings, and lowering body fat percentages. When doing moderate intensity exercise such as aerobic conditioning, fat is the primary energy source used by the body for fuel. So this is a good fat-burning activity.

Strength Training. Strength training or isotonic exercise enhances the muscle's ability to exert force against moveable resistance that produces muscle strength and stimulates muscle growth or size. Isometric (forcing against an immovable object) and isokenetic exercises, negative resistance training, floor or free-hand exercises (gravity training), and manual resistance exercises are good examples of strength training. Multi-station exercise machines, conventional cables and pulleys with weight stacks, plate-loaded equipment and handy free weights such as barbells or dumbbells are all tools of the trade for strength training.

Strength training shapes and tones muscles as well as making them stronger. Strength training helps elevate your good cholesterol (HDL) levels, which in turn contributes to lowering bad cholesterol (LDL). Strength training stimulates your metabolic rate for burning fat calories. Strength training also aids in the prevention of injury by promoting proper balance among the various muscle groups.

Flexibility Training. This type of training enhances and promotes the ability to move a joint through the full range of motion (ROM) without discomfort. Full range of motion for every joint is a must for healing, restoring, and developing proper joint action.

||||||||||||||||||||||||||||| **HEALTHY TIP** ||||||||||||||||||||||||||||

Three Components of an Exercise Program
1. Aerobic conditioning
2. Strength training
3. Flexibility training

Static stretching is a form of stretching that gently promotes elongation and flexibility of muscle and soft tissue. It is best to stretch the muscle until it becomes comfortably tight, but not painfully tight. Then hold that position for approximately 15 to 30 seconds. Release the stretch and take the muscle back to its original position.

This form of stretching does not involve any ballistic or bouncing motion. Do not jerk the limbs you are stretching, but simply apply a constant, gentle stretch. Be careful not to stretch beyond that comfort point, or you will not be able to relax the muscle; therefore, you will not benefit from the stretching exercise. Repeat this procedure four to six times per muscle group as well as every time you feel the need to stretch. Make sure you breathe deeply and slowly for a better stretch.

The benefits from stretching and flexibility exercises are a decrease in muscle and joint injury and soreness and the lengthening of muscle and connective tissue. Stretching will reduce stress, reduce joint pain, and increase your ability to relax.

|||||||||||||||||||||||||| **HEALTHY TIP** ||||||||||||||||||||||||||

Setting Goals

What are your goals? Be sure they are:

- Precise, simple, and obtainable
- Short-term
- Specific to your body condition

||||||||||||||||||||||||||||||||||||||||||||||||||||||||||||||||||||||||||

I prefer to see people warm up the muscles first then stretch them out. For example, the next time you decide to jog or power walk, it would be wise to walk gently for about ten minutes. Warm up those muscles by getting some blood pumping into them and some sinew fluid flowing in the joints. Then, after the short warm-up session, take time to stretch the muscles involved in your workout for that session.

Properly stretched muscles will perform at their optimum. Golfing, bowling, tennis, hiking, dancing, chasing the kids around—everything will become easier when your muscles are flexible.

SETTING FITNESS GOALS

Every time I present a seminar or workshop on exercise, I spend time afterward with a few people who are serious about getting back in shape. The problem is that most of them want to make a quantum leap from their current condition (one that took 20 years of abuse or neglect to produce) to their goal. It would be nice if we didn't have to climb a ladder one rung at a time to get to the top, but that is the safest and surest way.

|||||||||||||||||||||||||| **HEALTHY TIP** ||||||||||||||||||||||||||

Many people like to measure their success by using their scale, but I prefer not to. The scale can only tell you how much gravity is pulling you down at the moment; it doesn't tell you the composition or quality of your weight. My suggestion is to throw out the scale and use one of the other measurements of success instead.

|||||||||||||||||||||||||||||||||||||||||||||||||||||||||||||||||||||||||||||||||||||||||||||||||||||||||||||||

Part of climbing that ladder is having goals. Over the years I have observed that people who decide to make physical fitness part of their lifestyle start with one or two basic goals in mind. Exercise and healthy eating should be part of your lifestyle, not a quick fix. So set lifestyle goals. It is more likely that you will reach your goals by chipping away at them rather than trying to swallow them in one big gulp.

My recommendation is to first use my 80/20 plan: if people make food selections compatible for their blood type 80 percent of the time, the remaining 20 percent will not disrupt their goals or health and will make them happier. The same goes for exercising. Instead of trying to max out on every exercise you do in the gym, try building up slowly week by week until you reach the goal.

If your goal is to lose four dress sizes, then set out to drop the first one. After you have reached that goal, go on to the next dress size. This tactic keeps you motivated because your short-range goals are being reached. If your goal is to build more muscle on your chest, you will be most apt to succeed if you make your goal to gain the first inch. Then set out for the next inch. This establishes a good foundation for success. Keep yourself around 80 percent of your maximum strength level.

Create a way to measure your performance when setting goals. I'll use as an example my wife, Lori, and two neighbors who walk three to four nights a week. They started out walking three miles in 60 minutes. To measure their performance, they bettered their time. Thirty days later, Lori and her friends finished the same three miles in 55 minutes, then another 30 days at 50 minutes, etc. Your performance can be measured by the decrease in time it takes you to walk three miles. That decrease in time indicates an increase in fitness.

Measuring your performance provides evidence of work being accomplished and gives you a means to evaluate your program. Remember, remaining motivated is the key.

Tools for Motivation and Success

The following are several tools that will help you and your body stay strong.

A fitness journal can monitor your journey to a healthier you. It is always a good idea to write down where you are throughout the process. As you successfully reach your goals, you will have a record of what you accomplished. In case you find yourself backsliding, a quick glimpse at your journal will help you get back on track. An example of a fitness journal with a complete DVD series can be found in my Fork in Road series. (Visit www.bodyredesigning.com.)

Write down your goals along with the method you have chosen of measuring your success. Include feedback and the rewards. Reviewing them from time to time reinforces your strategy and your motivation.

Remember, some people enjoy using journals as a tool; others don't. I recommend them in the beginning to help you get started and stay on track. Later you may not need one to remain on track. Then you will instinctively know when to push yourself more.

Body fat testing and retesting have proven to be very helpful tools for monitoring success and providing evidence that you are accomplishing your goal. There are a few different ways to test your body fat. One is with the use of calipers, which are instruments used by a personal trainer, exercise physiologist, or specially trained person to take a reading of the thickness of your skin folds at various sites on your body.

Another method of testing body fat is an impedance machine that measures the resistance or time an electrical signal takes to travel through the body. This machine prints out the data that shows your body fat percentage and weight, your muscle weight, and the percentage of water in the tissue.

These tests are safe, pain-free, harmless, and can be performed at your local YMCA or health club. Chart these measurements so you can follow your progress on a regular basis.

Feedback is most helpful when trying to stay focused on your goals. How many times has just a single word of positive affirmation been just the push you needed to continue?

||||||||||||||||||||||||||||||||**HEALTHY TIP**||||||||||||||||||||||||||

Tools for Exercise Success

1. A fitness journal
2. Body fat testing and retesting
3. Feedback
4. Accountability
5. Rewards

||||||||||||||||||||||||||||||||||||||||||||||||||||||||||||||||||||||||||||||||||||||||||

Accountability is having someone who keeps you accountable. This person gives you the compliments and encouragement to help you stay focused. As you stay focused and committed to giving it your best effort, others will say positive things about you as well. Besides the compliments from others, the positive way you feel about yourself and the progress you see will be wonderful feedback for you.

Rewards await you as you press on to success. Your reward could be fitting into some of those beautiful clothes that you haven't been able to wear for months or maybe a shopping spree to purchase an entirely new wardrobe to replace that sport jacket and slacks that shrunk in the closet. Every time you reach an intermediate or short-term goal, consider rewarding yourself. Don't worry; you won't spoil yourself. But getting rewards every month can certainly help you stay committed.

Remember you will have some plateaus to hurdle; there will be times when you won't see any progress, and you'll feel like quitting because you think you'll never reach your goals. Do not allow negative thoughts to enter your mind. Stay positive, stay the course, and always remember—you are an inspiration in transition to others and yourself.

RENEWING YOUR MIND

- Reduce pent-up stress: pray, meditate, practice belly breathing.

- Stabilize blood sugar levels; protein aids in regulating carbohydrates/blood sugar by slowing down the conversion or burning off of glucose.

- Reduce cholesterol: diet, increase fiber in diet.

- Reduce pain levels: stretching, massage, positive thinking, reduction in stress.

- Enhance energy and vitality.

- Make selections for your blood type to accurately re-nourish your muscles.

- Hydrate before and after workouts to remove muscle wastes and for cellular health.

CHAPTER 29

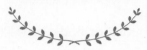

REDESIGNING YOUR BODY

*"Body redesigning is all about using your body
genetics for reaching your goals!"* —DR. JOE

When you see an infomercial on television that shows a couple of fitness models demonstrating a piece of exercise equipment, you receive the message to get your body into great shape. Body shaping or redesigning can definitely be a benefit of exercise, but it requires consideration of body type, blood type, genetics, health issues, and physical limitations.

BODY TYPES

How is it that someone you know (and we all do know a person like this) can eat anything he or she desires and never put on a pound? Then there are people like us—we simply look at food and our pants tighten up. By understanding how genetic factors play a huge role in the success of your fitness efforts, you will be less likely to get discouraged and give up. Through proper application of the right exercise methodology for your genetics, you will experience greater success with less pressure and guilt, and you will reach your genetic potential.

It is estimated that 75 percent of our body typing comes straight from our genes. So the pressure is on your parents and their parents and their parents—not you! Heredity is not totally responsible for our shapes, because each one of us can do things to improve the not-so-perfect body we have been given.

If there is a true category of body types (and the jury is still out on this one), the questions are: What am I working with? What are my bodily attributes? What works best for my body type?

Perhaps you have an apple-shaped body, with most of your weight in your upper body. To create a balanced physique, you would have to build up your lower body—the legs. But if you have a pear-shaped body, with most of the weight in the hips and thighs, you would not want to perform those bulk-building lower body exercises. Instead, you would do exercises that fill out your upper body. However, if you have a banana-shaped body, then adding curves to your body will work best. The body type with which you were born must be factored into your fitness program if you want to have specific results.

Before I go any further, I want to make sure you understand that when I am talking about redesigning the body, I am referring exclusively to the physical body. Far too often people confuse their physical condition or appearance with the person on the inside! Remember, the body is only the compartment that houses the real you.

BODY TYPES AND EXERCISE

Before I list the body types, their characteristics, and exercise prescriptions, I must remind you that it is impossible to restructure your musculoskeletal system. In other words, if you have short clavicles (the bones that give your shoulders their width), but you desire wide shoulders, forget about it. If your hip bone measures 35 inches and you want 30-inch hips, it's not going to happen. These are predisposed genetic traits that make up your body.

But don't close the book yet. There is still hope! Through exercise, you can take your body's genetically given structure to a level of shapeliness and new curves that did not come with the package. You cannot outsmart your genes, but you can use exercise strategies that are compatible with them.

These textbook body types may not describe you perfectly. As you examine yourself and your family members, you might discover that there is a little of each morph in your shape and size. But your body probably tends to have more characteristics of one over the others.

So, let's begin with the most traditional categories of body classifications. Is your body type an endomorph, an ectomorph, or a mesomorph?

The Endomorph

Endomorphic body types are people with bulky bodies. If your body type is an endo, then your main concentration should be losing body fat. Cardiovascular training works best for you. You should spend about 70 percent of your training time doing aerobic sessions. Up to 30 percent of your time should be in strength training. For the rest, do some form of stretching or flexibility training.

Aerobic training. Stay away from group fitness classes that conduct high-impact aerobics. Stay with low-impact exercises such as walking on the treadmill or riding a stationary bike.

Strength training. Concentrate on the large muscle groups (chest, back, arms, shoulders, and legs) and keep the repetitions high and the weights moderate.

Flexibility training. Center your focus on stretching classes to strengthen the hips and the knees.

The Ectomorph

The ectomorphic body type is the thinnest of all the body shapes. Ectos come with a stingy genetic disposition that fights against weight gain. For some it's a blessing; for others it's a curse. If this is your type, then special attention should be given not to overtrain. This body type will easily tap into its cellular reserves for muscle growth, repair or energy if the workout is too intense. My recommendation is to spend approximately 80 percent of training sessions on muscle stimulation through strength training. Spend about 10 percent on cardiovascular training and 10 percent on stretching and flexibility training.

Aerobic training. Keep it to a minimum. Try stationary biking or using a treadmill, an eclipse or any preferred cardio workout. Keep the time between 10 to 12 minutes. The best time for this is after your workout or on your off days.

Strength training. Every ecto should place most of the focus on strength training. To properly train, the ecto should use the heaviest weights possible for every exercise, while keeping the repetitions down to six or eight.

Ideally, ectos, with their fast metabolism, need only take each exercise to positive failure in order to stimulate their muscles to grow. In a pushing-type exercise, the pushing away of the weight from the body is the positive side, and the lowering or returning of the weight is the negative side. Positive failure occurs when an exercise cannot go any further than the last rep in the positive side of the exercise. Ectos should use a weight that will not allow them to go past six or eight reps, not even by one rep. That means using as much weight as possible. Keep the sets at three to four. Train one body part every five to six days.

Flexibility training. Concentrate on the major muscle groups—the lower and upper back, shoulders, arms, quadriceps (frontal thigh muscles), and hamstrings (rear thigh muscles). This is important for strengthening the joints.

The Mesomorph

If you have a mesomorphic body type, then genetically speaking you have been blessed with the ideal body type. Mesos have a naturally well-balanced, symmetrical physique and therefore can focus on their goals instead of concentrating on exercises that make up for their body type. Mesos respond very well to any exercise. They have a natural ability to build muscle weight easily with symmetrical balance.

Aerobic training and Strength training. Split your training up between these two.

Flexibility training. Stretch the major muscle groups. Flexibility is necessary for joint strength.

Along with information for the body morphs just described, try incorporating the following body shape guidelines. Use them as a starting point, but experiment until you find what fits you best.

BODY SHAPES

For years physiologists have used the apple and pear metaphors to help classify body shapes. Males are usually the classic apple shape, notorious for gaining weight around their upper torsos and midsections. Females are generally pear-shaped, storing most of their excess body fat on their thighs and hips. But my 30-plus years of observation have proven that women in particular are typed as being either a pear, an apple or a banana.

The easiest way to determine your body type is by answering the following question: If I gain weight, where does most of it go?

- If you answer hips, thighs and buttocks, you are a pear.

- If you answer stomach, arms and back, you are an apple.

- If you answer both upper and lower, you are a banana.

When I was involved in the pageant industry, helping the women prepare for the swimsuit competition, I saw amazing and dramatic results from exercise. The majority of the female body types I worked with were the true pear shape. I recall one young woman in particular who had very large hips, thighs and buttocks, a small waist, a flat bust line and narrow shoulders.

At the end of 90 days of training, she had dropped five inches off her thighs, hips and buttocks areas. She had also added two inches to her bust measurement and her shoulder measurement. Her figure had gained the most pleasing symmetry that her body type would allow. Her body went from the genetic pear-shaped figure of 34-25-41 to a redesigned symmetrical 36-24-36.

Of course, her motivation and commitment level were extremely strong because of the competition. But this level of commitment is common once people identify their genetic structure and apply the proper exercise methodology.

We always want to place more emphasis on the weaker areas to bring them up to par with the stronger ones. This altering of your appearance will not change your genetic baseline, but it will bring out your genetic potential.

Remember, let your fitness condition—not the program—dictate how much exercise to do. If you are unfit, then start slowly and work up to the optimum exercises.

Apples

Aerobic sessions. Try treadmill, stair climbing, and cycling. These sessions should be short in duration and high in intensity. Build up to 30 minutes at about 65 percent of your maximum heart rate. Of course, this must be adjusted to your present physical fitness condition.

Cardiovascular interval training sessions. During a 20 to 25 minute workout, vary the intensity every few minutes. Exercise at 65 percent of your maximum heart rate for five minutes, then drop down to 60 percent again for the next five minutes. Continue varying the intensity for the whole workout.

Strength training (redesigning). Concentrate on the upper torso, specifically on your shoulders, chest and upper back. Keep the repetitions between 10 and 12, and perform three sets per exercise per body part. Start off at 20 to 25 minutes per workout.

Because you are heavy on the top and taper down at the hips and thighs, you should concentrate on heavy lower body exercises. Try incorporating squats, leg presses, and calf raises. Do upper body exercises just for firming and toning the abs and pectorals.

Pears

Aerobic sessions. Try walking, cycling, and the treadmill. Your aerobic training sessions are nearly opposite to those for your fruitful friend, the apple. The intensity level is low, which means you can train for a longer duration. Aerobic training done for a long period of time will help metabolize fat storage. The length of your aerobic session is an individual thing, but go for a minimum of 30 minutes. You can work up to 45 minutes or 60 minutes if you are advanced and want to make significant improvements. Anything longer is not as productive.

Cardiovascular interval training sessions. During a 20 to 30 minute workout, vary the intensity every few minutes. Exercise at 65 percent of your maximum heart rate for five minutes, then drop down to 60 percent again for the next five minutes. Continue varying the intensity for the whole workout. This will speed up your metabolism.

Strength training (redesigning). Focus on the chest, shoulders, and arms. The repetitions should be eight to ten per set, with three sets per exercise per body part. This session should last up to 25 minutes.

Because your body is heavy at the hips, thighs, and buttocks, avoid completely any exercises that will bulk the muscles in the lower body. This includes any compound movements such as leg presses, squats, or power deadlifts.

Also avoid the stair-climbing machines and high-resistance stationary bike riding. Try isolation movements like high-rep, 90-degree, side leg lifts (hydrants) and iso-lunges. A hips isolation machine is excellent for targeting the hips and buttocks area. Also ride a stationary bike at low resistance.

Bananas

Aerobic sessions. Try walking, stair climbing, and cycling. You will want to keep the intensity low, allowing for a longer session. This aerobic session is done on your "off" days from your body redesigning workouts. Ideally, you should exercise from 30 minutes and build up to 45 minutes. This will assist your body in losing excess body fat.

Cardiovascular interval training sessions. During a 20 to 25 minute workout, vary the intensity every few minutes. Keeping the intensity from dropping too low is best. But exercising at 65 percent of your maximum heart rate for five minutes or so and then dropping down to 60 percent for five more is a good mix. You will want to stimulate your metabolism.

Strength training (redesigning). Because your genetics typically lack curves, building muscle (lean not bulky) on the upper and lower body work best. Focus equally on the upper and lower body with compound exercises for the lower body such as bench squats, deep-knee bends or weighted lunges, and weighted exercises for the upper body such as dumbbell chest press, around-the-world for shoulders and tricep/bicep dumbbell exercises. Of course, as with all body types, you will want to include abdominal exercises such as reverse crunches, twists, and regular crunches. This session should go for 20 to 25 minutes.

Because your body type is such that your upper and lower body are equal or straight up and down, then you are not as concerned with balancing your body's shape as you are with adding curves. By placing emphasis on reducing the waistline, broadening the shoulders, and adding curves to your hips, this can be accomplished.

POST-OP REHAB AND MORE!

I realize it is difficult to feel like exercising when you are in physical pain, haven't exercised for months (or ever) and particularly coming off a surgical procedure. But what will make all the difference in the world to you and your body is to take on a new attitude about your life. A change of perspective about living without pain or physical limitations should be your top priority. So let's take a peek at what you can and should consider doing after surgery.

If you had hip or knee replacement surgery or shoulder, foot, elbow or back surgery, etc. or any combination of them, you must participate in rehabilitating your joints, muscles, ligaments and tendons so you can get back on your feet (literally) and start living life anew!

The first line of recovery will be post-op rehabilitation. Immediately after surgery and while recovering in the hospital from surgery, your doctor may order the PT (physical therapist) to start a minor rehabilitation program until you are discharged from the hospital. Please be willing to do your best to follow his or her directions so you can prevent future problems. I know those who refused to go through rehabilitation and consequently required many more months to function normally than if they had participated in the rehab program. There where many others who started experiencing new pain or walked with a limp and even had difficulty in doing everyday tasks.

Whether you decide to go to a rehabilitation center or have a PT come to your home for post-op rehab, please be willing to allow them to do their job which in turn will make recovery and back to life again a smooth and enjoyable experience.

What to do after post-op rehab!

First and foremost, listen to your body. Your body is still weak and sore and limited to doing what a healthy body can do, so go slowly! Use some of the exercise ideas I listed in this book and or hire a personal trainer who is qualified to help post-op rehab patients rebuild their body.

It is important to exercise the whole body which will involve; weights, machines, stretch bands, etc and lots and lots of stretching exercises. It will be key to strengthen the muscles and ligaments/tendons that support your joints but also very important to stretch your joints to improve maximum ROM (range of motion).

Remember your post-op rehab program which may last 6 weeks or so is the initial step to recovery but an exercise program following your rehab program is more than a temporary program – it should become a part of your lifestyle which will lead to a new pain-free and healthy life......I know first hand!

I survived 2 emergency back surgeries and 2 complete hip replacements surgeries. In 2012 I had a second major back surgery on the L2, L3, L4 and L5 lumbar joints and in November 2013 and January 2014 I had complete hip replacement surgeries. So I know what it feels like to be in excruciating and crippling pain and being handicapped and helpless. But on the other hand I know what it feels like to leave that dreadful and painful season and rise above it as I am walking into this new season of rejuvenation, restoration and rebuilding.

I followed all the instructions from my PT for post-op rehab then I began my own strengthening program which has been taking baby steps at a time to where I am almost at 100% total function and enjoying life that was stolen from me for years and years by chronic pain.

I want to encourage you, if you value life (a gift from above), if you have reasons for living (loved ones, etc) then step up and make regular exercise a part of your life for the rest of your life – you will be glad you did!

RENEWING YOUR MIND

- Participate in Post-Op Rehab.
- Start an exercise program – hire a knowledgeable personal trainer.
- Exercise is NOT a form of punishment.
- Make regular exercise a lifetime commitment.
- Set specific goals, go at it slowly but surely.
- Enjoy your new pain-free and healthy life.

STEP 7

REST AND RELAXATION

CHAPTER 30

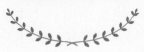

THE IMPORTANCE OF R&R

"It's not having time to relax but rather not knowing how to relax, that's the problem!" —Dr. Joe

Stress results from your body reaction to one or more stressors. There are physiological changes that occur when an individual is under stress. For example, arteries narrow, the heart beats faster and pumps blood harder, blood pressure elevates, blood sugar rises, and the body starts to sweat. Stress can cause flare-ups in chronic pain patients, weaken the immune system, and when chronic can lead to cancer, heart disease, and diabetes.

I could go on and on about the negative effects stress has on our bodies and minds, but I would rather help you by having you understand that it isn't so much what type of stressors you are dealing with but rather and most importantly, how you cope with stress. Sometimes even a very difficult situation that is stressful can be less harmful to your health if you change the way you look at the circumstance. Instead of looking at it fearfully, look at it as a challenge with a soon-to-be-found solution.

As I struggled with a painful condition, I put off hip replacement surgery in hopes of finding alternative medicine and practices that would heal my root causes rather than just cutting away parts and pieces of my body. In fact, I looked hopefully into the future while walking through my healing using many of the modalities, treatments, and other natural ways to heal my body. In the end I have found that my level of stress from dealing with pain day in and day out was less wearing as I refocused my mind from the dark side to a bright and hopeful ending and purpose.

JAMAICA

One year after my emergency lower back surgery, Lori and I were married in front of a tall waterfall at the Enchanted Gardens resort in Jamaica. We stayed at this island paradise, tucked away on the side of a mountain, for the most relaxing two weeks of my life.

Engulfed in tropical plants and flowers and abundant natural waterfalls and streams, we spent most of the time lounging around the heart-shaped pool listening to the steel drums of a Caribbean band. Sometimes we floated on rafts and let the sight of the tall, swaying palm trees put us to sleep.

But the most restful spot on the entire resort was right near our condo. I spotted it one day while walking over a little wooden bridge. There it was—a hammock stretched between two trees right next to the stream.

Eagerly, I slipped into it. The hypnotic sounds of water trickling over the rocks and birds chirping in the trees together with the steady swaying of the hammock put me right to sleep. The time I spent in that hammock really revived my overworked body and mind.

Whenever I think of rest and relaxation, those two blissful weeks of romance and nature come to mind.

We all like the idea of resting and relaxing. But do we know their value? We are so overcharged and revved up all the time that the very idea of leaving all our deadlines for a three-day R&R weekend can make us crazy!

Yet even our Creator took the seventh day to rest. I'm not sure He was actually fatigued or burned out from the preceding six days of creating the world. Nevertheless, Yahweh gave us a model—Sabbath Rest! So *make time to rest and relax!*

RELAXING BODY AND MIND

Rest is needed by our bodies to recover from physical stressors or even work, exercising, recreational activities, and everyday tasks. Our minds need rest from emotional stressors too, such as family situations, marriage relationships, financial woes, and employment or business concerns.

Rest and relaxation are absolutely necessary for rejuvenation. How long has it been since you got away by yourself and spent time recharging your emotional and spiritual batteries? Resting the body is essential for healing the body, bodily functions, and a tranquil mind. For me, resting, especially in the tropics with all the exotic sights and sounds, causes me to appreciate life and the Life Giver.

THE OVERLOAD ZONE

Most of us today live with so much stress and busyness that it often takes a major jolt to get our attention. If you have reached the point where life is no fun anymore, then you just might be held hostage to the Overload Zone. You end up in the Overload Zone when you get totally drained emotionally, physically, and spiritually.

|||||||||||||||||||||||||||||| **HEALTHY TIP** ||||||||||||||||||||||||||||||

Are You in the Overload Zone?

- Do you lack quality time with your spouse?
- Are you too preoccupied to fine-tune your marriage?
- Do you spend little or no time with your children?
- Do you lack sound sleep?
- Do you lack quiet time, prayer, and meditation?
- Do other people irritate you?
- Are your eating habits out of control?
- Do you lack regular exercise?
- Do you lack libido/sexual desire with your spouse?

- Are you spent and feel run-down and fatigued?

Once you hit the Overload Zone, your work performance suffers. Your family life becomes more like a second job, than a haven from the outside world, and your spiritual life has gone from a state of peace and tranquility to unsettled frustration.

Before it's too late, take a minute or two to see if you can identify with any of the Overload Zone symptoms. If you identified with one to three of these symptoms, you need some fine-tuning. If you identify with four to six of them, you need a minor overhaul. If seven or more sounded too familiar to you, a major overhaul is the only thing that will save your downhill slide.

Stop right now! Take a deep breath, hold it, and slowly let it through tight lips! In fact, do that again, two more times. Make immediate plans for rest and relaxation, then address each area with which you identified. I'll show you how.

STRESS—THE MODERN EPIDEMIC

If you scored high on the Overload Zone questions, then you need to de-stress. An overworked brain and an unused heart are typical red flags for stress. Progressive relaxation, a combined form of physical and emotional de-stressing, can help the brain and heart gradually return to their natural rhythms.

Think about it for a minute. How long has it been since you took a step back from your maddening pace to determine if your brain is overworked? If you are like most people who spend hours on the Internet, Facebook, etc., researching or just browsing every day, your brain can get overloaded with information and you can easily become mentally stressed.[1] Because of the overwhelming amount of information available to us today, we can easily become brain tired without realizing it.

During any given day we find ourselves confronted with various forms of stress. If you live in this modern world, I hardly need to name them for you. Traffic, relationships, chronic pain, poor health, finances—these and more are responsible for anxiety in our lives.

Hans Seyle, often called the father of stress studies, is a pioneer in stress research. The kinds of stress I named in the previous paragraph are negative stressors, which he calls distress. But on the other hand, there are positive stressors, which he calls eustress, or good stress.[2]

By adding more eustress, or good stress, into our lives on a daily basis, our lives can become more balanced.

HEALTHY TIP

De-Stressing

The three stages of de-stressing:

1. Identify the stress.
2. Examine the stress to determine the root cause.
3. Develop a stress management program that includes:

    Alternative creative solutions to deal with the stress

    Action steps you will take to manage the stress

    A way to record your progress

Here are a few eustress ideas to de-stress, but remember to be creative:

- Regularly add a 30-minute workout or walk followed by some form of stretching to your routine.

- Get a full body massage, one per month.

- Practice deep breathing exercises daily.

- Laugh more. Hang around people with good humor, often.

- Think positively, reject negative thoughts.

Creating harmony in our body and mind is directly linked to the way we balance the distress and the eustress in our lives. Unfortunately, living in a fast-paced society tends to keep us out of balance.

If you think you don't have time for eustress, then let me remind you that it is much easier to maintain your health than to try to repair it. Continued stress weakens the immune system, causes painful flare-ups and taxes the cardiovascular system, etc.

Less negative stress in our lives would be wonderful, but in a world as fast paced as ours, that is only part of the solution. Coping with the attitude we have toward stressful events is the important thing. It has been said, "Life is 10 percent how we make it, 90 percent how we take it." In and of itself, stress is not the problem; it's our perception of the situation that makes the difference. One person's dreaded family reunion is another person's picnic. We can deliberately change our way of thinking about a stressful situation so that its negative effect on us is reduced. It takes a little effort, but it is worth it.

Perhaps you arrive home from work stressed from not only the workload, but also from office politics, pettiness, and unfairness. If there is someone at home to talk to about your day, then you can get things off your chest. After a while, you will feel calmer. Perhaps you can even laugh at some of the things that made you uptight during the day. You remember together that life doesn't always run smoothly. Even having a pet helps relieve stress after a long, hard day.

Once mentally relieved by the talk, it's a good idea to do something to de-stress physically, too. Perhaps taking a walk or enjoying a soak in the tub will help to bring down your blood pressure and heart rate.

Once you start noticing when you are stressed, take the measures that work for you personally to remove the stress from your life.

A first step in de-stressing is identifying the source or sources of stress. What causes you the most stress? A person at work, your boss, your children's friends, finances, your chronic pain, etc. The goal is to identify the source(s) of stress.

Determine the root cause. Is it emotional, mental, or physical? Why is this event particularly stressful for you? Maybe you have an emotional wound in a certain area that is pricked by the person at the office or by your boss. Perhaps you fear failing financially because that happened to your parents and you lived through it. Or maybe it's just a character flaw you need to accept and deal with, such as a bad temper or sharp tongue. Understanding the root of the stress will aid you in changing your perspective toward it.

Once you have determined the root of your stress, you can create alternative ways of coping with it. For instance, I could be an impatient driver, particularly when it came to someone driving while texting or the other way around. I could feel myself getting all jacked up over this person in front of me who had no idea of where his car was on the road or that the red light turned green two minutes ago or he was driving way under the speed limit. After experiencing pain in my shoulders and neck as well as elevated blood pressure, I decided to change my perspective. Because it is impossible to change the way others drive, I decided to slow down, even leave earlier for my appointments. I am now able to laugh at the situation and don't let it stick to me. And with a few deep breaths and good music on, driving has become less stressful.

I identified the stressful event—driving. My impatience was the root of my stress. By changing my perspective toward drivers who aren't paying attention while driving, I now drive with much less stress.

Changing our stressful habits can really aid us in reducing tension in our lives. But we also need to actively practice positive techniques such as progressive relaxation to de-stress.

RENEWING YOUR MIND

- Take time to slow down and chill out.
- Turn the world off at various times when stress is mounting.
- Do belly breathing daily.
- Eat foods compatible with your blood type for accuracy.
- Laugh more, play more, and forgive yourself more.
- Have more sex with your spouse—it's very healthy!

CHAPTER 31

PROGRESSIVE RELAXATION

*"Laugh more, do fun things and remember life is short enough,
it doesn't need your help to make it shorter!"* —DR. JOE

Stress management activities should be part of our everyday lives. They reduce the level of anxiety and emotional distress we may be experiencing and help us release the negative buildup that contributes to chronic pain flare-up, weakening our immune system, and basically destroying our health.

As you get relief using the following techniques, I hope you will incorporate them into your daily life, because they will help you feel good and have much more energy. Consider spending some time—in the mornings before you start your day or at night after the kids are in bed—doing these stress relievers so you can start your day off right or get a good night's sleep.

DEEP BREATHING

As I mentioned earlier in the book, I first started practicing this technique to improve my mental imagery for perfecting the squat back in my power lifting days. But today it is custom-made for channeling my stress and anxieties. Because stressful situations are directly linked to our physical responses, it behooves us to make this breathing exercise part of our daily life. It will bring you stress relief!

Find a comfortable position on the floor or in a chair and allow your body to go limp (while sitting upright). Then force yourself to inhale slowly for as long as you can from the belly. Fill your belly full of air and hold it for a second, then slowly exhale all the air out of your lungs through your tightly held lips. Aim for one slow inhale and one slow exhale every minute, forcing all the air out of your lungs each time.

Don't be disappointed if you cannot make one cycle of breathing last 60 seconds. You will most likely have to build up to it, but in the process you will learn how to relax your body at will. Try this breathing exercise for five minutes at a time.

This breathing technique will help reduce your blood pressure, heart rate and pulse, plus it will calm the muscles that are tight from tension and stress.

This relaxation exercise will be very beneficial to you, particularly if you have speaking engagements, an interview for a job or a salary increase, or just need to slow things down in the middle of the day. It will put your body and mind in a very calming mood.

After you master this breathing technique, it won't matter where you are because you can do it anywhere, anytime.

MUSCLE TENSING

Muscle tension from physical exertion is one thing but when our muscles are tense due to stress, then our entire bio-chemistry changes, which can be manifested in elevated blood pressure, nervousness, headaches, etc.

When we tense our muscles for a few moments and then release them, our body responds by relaxing, de-stressing, and offers a more calm state of mind and body. Make time to do the following routine when you feel life is getting too much to handle. It doesn't matter what is stressing you out but rather finding natural and healthy ways to de-stress. It's a great stress management exercise!

||||||||||||||||||||||||||**HEALTHY TIP**||||||||||||||||||||||||||||

Order of muscle groups to tense:[1]

- Clench your right fist. This relaxes the right hand and forearm.
- Clench your left fist. This relaxes the left hand and forearm.
- Clench both fists.
- Bend both wrists.
- Frown. This relaxes the forehead and scalp.
- Squint your eyes. This relaxes the eye and face muscles.
- Clench your teeth. This relaxes the jaw.
- Push back against the headrest. This relaxes the neck.
- Shrug your shoulders. This relaxes the shoulders and back.
- Take a deep breath. Hold it, then forcefully exhale. This relaxes the chest.
- Tighten your abdominal (stomach) muscles.
- Tighten your buttocks, thighs, and calves all at once. This relaxes the lower extremities.
- Point your toes forward. This relaxes the foot muscles.

Muscle tensing can bring relaxation to our bodies, too. Called progressive muscle relaxation, this process is simply working with one muscle group at a time by tensing the muscle for eight to ten seconds and then releasing the tension. You will feel the tension leave as you do this. Try to perform these exercises when nobody is around to interrupt the session. You can sit while you do these exercises. If you prefer to lie on the floor, roll up a towel and place it under your neck for support. Each session should last about 10-14 minutes.

Prepare for your session by getting comfortable. Take off your shoes and loosen your belt and tie—or remove them. Remove your glasses or contacts if you wear them. Then close your eyes and relax the best you can (the breathing technique can help here) for a minute or two. Then take the following steps:

1. Working with one muscle group at a time, tense each muscle group two times for 15 seconds each time. Do it in the order listed in the Healthy Tip box. Move at a slow pace.

2. Pause and take deep breaths intermittently.

3. Contract your muscles at approximately 60 to 70 percent of maximum output, or until they are fairly tight.

When you are finished, take a deep breath. Hold, then forcefully exhale. As you exhale say, "Relax." This mental reinforcement improves your concentration and helps you relax even more. Rest for two to three minutes, then get up.

I know some of the de-stressing exercises may seem nonsensical and somewhat ridiculous to do. But if you are in pain, if you are finding it difficult to cope with life because of getting weary from being overstressed and experiencing many painful sleepless nights, it may be these simple but very efficacious exercises that will see you through.

We all have various stressful situations that we have to cope with in our daily lives. There is no doubt when you have to cope with a chronic painful joint or painful condition it doesn't take much to cause you to become stressed out. We do not have to be victims of the Overload Zone, and we certainly do not have to rely on medications to calm us down when we are capable of doing some simple but productive exercises that can help us wind down and de-stress.

As you relax and practice those deep belly breathing exercises or unwinding with the muscle tension exercises, you can mentally go to a white sandy beach of a tropical island or float in the warm ocean listening to steel drums to help you relax even further. That peaceful hammock in Jamaica does the trick for me!

RENEWING YOUR MIND

- Stress can be managed. It is a matter of coping with your stress so to avoid the damaging effects it can have on your overall health.

- A blood type compatible diet is the essential baseline for stress.

- Healthy sexual relations with your spouse will do wonders for stress.

- Take up a hobby, recreation, etc.

- Practice breathing exercises.

- Exercise regularly.

- Listen to relaxing music.

- Start laughing again. Find those funny people who make you laugh and invite them over to the house.

- Pray, mediate, and count your blessings.

CHAPTER 32

A GOOD NIGHT'S REST

*"There's nothing you can do about tomorrow's problems
when you go to bed so lights out!"* —DR. JOE

The average person spends about one-third of his or her life asleep. That might sound like a waste of a lot of good hours! You could be doing something more productive—golfing, training, or making a buck, right? No, sleep is actually productive time because your body regenerates itself through sleep.

REBUILDING YOUR HEALTH THROUGH SLEEP

Whether you are always pushing the envelope, high stung, and an overachiever or you are calm and have your life in balance, there is one common denominator between the two personalities—a good night's sleep.

Yet both lifestyles, when pushed to the limit, can stress the body and shortchange its health. Our bodies are capable of handling just so much physical work and mental and emotional strain. Then they need to recharge with a good night's sleep. Those precious hours under the covers are exactly what our body needs for optimum efficiency.

Your nighttime sleeping patterns can be disrupted by living in the Overload Zone for too long. Too much stress, constant anxiety, and poor dietary habits can interfere with a good night's sleep. Actually, even doing good things such as physical exercise or training can interfere with your deep-sleep patterns. The more intense your workouts, the more adjustments your body has to make.

Research shows that sleeping every night is one of the most important things we can do for our health. While we are sleeping, not doing much in the way of activity, our bodies are hard at work repairing and rebuilding. During sleep, at a specific time, the body produces and releases hormones and neurotransmitters to repair and rebuild itself. Generally, this time is when the individual reaches rapid-eye movement (REM) sleep. But if REM is not reached, then these metabolic processes are interrupted, and a breakdown in health begins.

As we already learned, building lean muscle weight is ideal for many reasons. But you will find it interesting that it is not during your workouts that your muscles grow. They actually grow while you sleep. The process of growth and repair of muscles is regulated by a number of neurotransmitters and hormones. The orchestra leader in charge of this biochemical band is melatonin.

MELATONIN

Melatonin, a hormone that is released by a tiny pea-sized gland in our brains called the pineal gland, is responsible for setting our internal clocks. The sleep-wake cycle is directly linked to the precise timing of the release of this hormone.

As our bodies age, they produce less melatonin, which causes them to no longer reach the deep state of sleep they did when they were younger. Reaching that deep-sleep state is necessary for the body to rebuild and repair itself.

The amount of deep sleep we get, along with the amount of melatonin that is released, affects the release of other biochemicals such as HGH (human growth hormone), DHEA, cortisol, and the steroid hormones. These hormones stimulate immune function, muscle growth, tissue repair, and a myriad of other essential processes.[1]

Our Creator saw fit to design and program His human creation to have their sleep-wake cycle coincide with day and night. Darkness is directly responsible for the release of melatonin, which peaks around 2 o'clock in the morning and returns to the baseline at approximately 8 a.m. The problem is we don't always listen to our bodies, so sometimes we don't get the sleep we need.

Have you ever pulled an all-nighter? Or stayed up until 1 or 2 a.m. checking your email, Facebook account, or watching a movie? Staying up all night creates a significant challenge to the immune system. Studies have shown that getting inadequate sleep can interfere with the normal release of HGH—and less HGH speeds up the aging process.

Over time, if you are not getting a full night's sleep for whatever reason, your body will start suppressing your melatonin secretions. This, in turn, plays havoc with your body's hormonal balance. When this pattern of being up all night becomes the rule instead of the exception, this sleep debt will eventually catch up with you. During the daytime, your reaction time will be slower, your brain will feel foggy, and you won't make good decisions. If you are not getting enough sleep, you will be sleepy and fatigued during the day. Most people think that drinking several cups of coffee does the trick. Sorry, that won't help. Your body is fatigued because you missed the sleep, not because you are caffeine depleted.

With this in mind, if you plan to buy a car anytime in the near future, remember not to buy one that was built on a Monday! All the weekend warriors and party animals are on the assembly line Monday morning, probably sleepy and fatigued from their weekends.

Missing sleep night after night will weaken your immune system. Before you realize it, you will have caught every bug that is flying around the office. Eventually this sleep debt may increase the chances of heart disease and development of osteoporosis because of the hormonal imbalance that results. You must get enough deep rest every night for good health.

DEVELOP GOOD SLEEPING HABITS

It's important to do whatever it takes to get a good night's rest. One of the things Lori and I do to protect our sleep is have our bedroom phone on mute. That way those rude and thoughtless telemarketers or wrong-number callers don't disrupt a good night's sleep.

Developing good sleeping habits starts with regularity. Going to bed at the same time each night and waking up at the same time each morning is ideal. I realize that may seem impossible, especially with the pace we keep in our Western culture. We tend to do all the wrong things for a good night sleep. We eat late at night. We drink caffein-ated beverages or alcohol, or food types with caffeine. We carry a load of mental problems and issues to bed instead of leaving them at our workplace. So instead of falling to sleep, we lie there going over the list of issues and problems and can't fall asleep. When it comes to going to bed to sleep, I have learned to talk to my brain. I simple tell it, "There is nothing I can do about such and such in bed so just go to sleep." And in seconds I'm sleeping.

Perhaps you have heard people say they are morning people or night people. What does a married couple do when one spouse is a night person and the other is a morning person? Lori and I are oppo-sites like that. She finds it difficult to go to bed before midnight, and I could go to bed at 10 p.m. She loves to sleep in, and I couldn't sleep in if my life depended on it. She needs something to stop her mind from thinking so she can fall asleep. I am asleep on the way down to the pillow. She will listen to her iPad in bed but watching TV to go to sleep is done in the theater—never in the bedroom. In the meanwhile, I'm in dreamland.

So, how can two people like us hit the hay at the same time?

I suggested she take melatonin at night before she wanted to go to bed. Melatonin is a powerful antioxidant and aids in deep sleep. Because our bodies produce less melatonin as we age, whether we exercise and eat healthy foods or not, I thought it a wise preventative practice to add to my daily dietary supplement regime. Lori started taking it too; one hour before she plans to go to bed, she takes melatonin. Then at bedtime, she finds herself ready for sleep. It works great!

You might want to consider adding this dietary supplementation to your new healthy lifestyle. Of course the dosages are different for different people, so I suggest you talk with a nutritional professional for advice. However, remember that melatonin is a powerful neuro-hormone that should not be used in a haphazard manner.[2]

INSOMNIA AND CHEMICAL COMPLICATIONS

One of the most aggravating frustrations that people can experience is insomnia—not being able to fall asleep, no matter how tired they are. Mental exercises, such as counting sheep or thinking in circles, only frustrate the problem. No wonder there are so many sleep medications prescribed for the non-sleeper.

Studies in sleep labs have shown that insomniacs need more time to enter the first stage of sleep than others do.[3] Additionally, often the REM state and the dream state of insomniacs are disrupted because of individuals' erratic sleeping patterns. They toss and turn, awakening frequently, and often arise feeling as though they had no rest.

Many insomniacs take sleeping pills, but sleeping medications can interfere with REM sleep, alter sleep patterns, and induce chemical dependency. Consequently, people who take these chemicals regularly may never be fully rested. Plus, after a period of time, the body builds immunity to the medications and requires more, thus creating problems of addiction.

Other people may drink alcohol to calm them down at the end of a busy day. But drinking alcohol before bedtime actually prevents a person from entering into REM sleep and can cause nighttime hypoglycemia, which is a very common cause for awakening at night.[4]

Perhaps you've heard a person who drank too much the night before say, "I slept like a log last night." Not a chance! REM sleep was never reached, so that person did not wake up the next morning fully rested. That's often obvious to everyone but the person speaking!

Another reason insomniacs find it hard to sleep is that they think they need more sleep than they actually require. Deep REM sleep is what is required for rest and recovery, not necessarily the old standard of eight to ten hours of any kind of sleep. In reality, what insomniacs need is better nutrition. The better the nutrition, through blood type compatible food selections and dietary supplements, the less sleep the body needs.

NATURAL SLEEP AIDS

Tests have shown that certain nutrients can induce and help maintain sleep. Nature has fascinating ways of helping our body repair, rebuild, relax, and rejuvenate without the use of medication or drugs. When used in their proper amounts, the following nutrients can be helpful for sleep.

Calcium plays an important role to calm nervousness and restlessness, thereby helping us sleep. Children who are hyperactive have been known to experience a calming effect from calcium supplementation. The best way to take calcium is with magnesium. Calcium and magnesium work most effectively in a dosage of two parts calcium to one part magnesium (2:1 ratio).

Magnesium plays a huge role in normalizing the activity of the nerves. It stores itself in the skeletal muscles and promotes the necessary stimuli for muscular control and relaxation. Magnesium also protects muscles from cramping.

Hops is regarded as a powerful, stimulating, and relaxing nerve tonic. It is good for cardiovascular disorders, yet it produces soothing rest for anxiety, hyperactivity, insomnia, nervousness, restlessness, and stress. Hops helps relax the liver and gall ducts, and even serves as a mild laxative. Some people find that placing it inside a pillowcase aids sleep.

Chamomile tea is a natural sedative. It is a traditional remedy for stress, anxiety, indigestion, and insomnia.

Holy Basil enhances the body's response to stress and the negative effects stress has on the body. Holy Basil also helps with the fear of flying as it calms the nervous system and allows the body to relax.

Alfalfa contains powerful trace minerals. It also contains vitamin A and enzymes that assist the body in digestion. It helps sleep indirectly by calming the digestive tract, also providing some relief from peptic ulcers, kidney and bladder problems, as well as pain relief from arthritis.

Inositol is a member of the B family and has been proven to help patients sleep.

Pantothenic acid is a member of the B vitamin family and works well with inositol for relaxation.

L-tryptophan is not a vitamin but an amino acid (one of nature's building blocks from which protein is made). Your body does not manufacture it, so you need to supplement it with your diet. L-tryptophan has an effect of feeling sleepy like after eating turkey meat.

Niacinamide is another member of the B vitamin family and enhances the effects of tryptophan.

When you experiment with natural dietary supplements as alternatives to pharmaceutical sleep inducers, you will find they work opposite from the drugs. Barbiturates prescribed for sleeping purposes usually start with lower dosages and must be increased as the body becomes addicted to the drugs.

But with dietary supplements, you might need to take heavier amounts at first in order to help get your body healthy and functioning properly. Then, after your body is healed and has improved bodily performance and function, the dosages often can be reduced to a minimum. In many cases, they won't be needed at all.

Anxiety is somewhat related to insomnia. The nutrients that are helpful for one are also helpful for the other.

SUPPLEMENTS TO FIGHT AGAINST PAIN AND SLEEPLESS NIGHTS

The importance of getting regular sleep cannot be stressed enough. Sleep deprivation leads to hormonal imbalance, which in turn disrupts the body's ability to repair itself and rebuild muscle tissue. Without sleep, the body cannot meet its other hormonal needs. Plus, the aging process is speeded up—and who wants that?

If you suffer from sleep deprivation or poor night sleep patterns because you have chronic, acute, arthritic pain, etc., you know how it wears you down over time. Your body and mind becomes tired throughout the day, it is difficult to concentrate. So with that in mind I have put together a list of common anti-inflammatory and arthritic pain dietary supplements that you may want to consider:

Allium sativum (garlic) has properties for reducing elevated cholesterol and works well for RA.

Boswellia serrata (shallaki) contains *boswellic acid* and works well for arthritis and RA.

Chondroitin sulphate helps rebuild cartilage and is a natural arthritis supplement.

Glucosamine is known to reduce arthritic-like pain and joint inflammation.

Commiphora mukul (guggulu) is a natural arthritis supplement.

Curcuma longa (haridra) is commonly known as *turmeric*. It is a powerful anti-inflammatory and helps relieve swelling in the joints.

Flax, Flaxseed Oil contain omega-3s and work well for RA and inflammatory problems. Both are very beneficial for constipation and colon health.

Harpagophytum procumbens (devil's claw), African herb that reduces pain and swelling of joints.

Methylsulfonylmethane (MSM), works well for arthritis and RA joints.

Omega-3 fatty acids; Omega-3 oil is derived from fish oil. As an anti-inflammatory supplement it works well for RA and other inflammatory conditions.

Trigonella foenum-graecum (fenugreek seed) works well for arthritis and muscular pain.

Zingiber officinale (ginger) works well for arthritis and RA.

As you reduce the level of pain that has been disrupting your sleep and life as a whole, supplementing your diet (foods for your blood type) with natural anti-inflammatory and arthritis pain nutrients, you will be able to reestablish your sleep-wake cycle. The payoffs: improved overall health, less pain, better recovery from stress, a strong immune system, and less anxiety.

(See Dr. Joe's Pain Management Nutrients, in the Resources section in the back of the book.)

RENEWING YOUR MIND

- Maintain a regular schedule for bedtime and waking.

- Create the right sleeping environment: dark room, very cool temperature with no electronics including TV.

- Go to bed for sex and sleep, nothing else.

- Pre-bedtime exercise: warm bath, read a book, listen to relaxing music, etc.

- Write down any problems or concerns and clear your mind of them.

- Eat three hours before bedtime, no caffeine, alcohol, chocolates, or soft drinks containing caffeine.

- Workouts should be completed four hours before bedtime.

- If you awake, lie there and relax. If you cannot fall back to sleep then get up and do something calming until you fall to sleep.

- Consider taking the nutritional supplements cited.

STEP 8

STRATEGIES FOR ANTI-AGING

CHAPTER 33

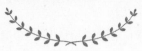

AGING AND DETERIORATION

"The goal is to die young—as late as possible." —ASHLEY MONTAGU

If you're reading this book, there's a good chance you are a baby boomer—an American born between 1946 and 1964. Baby boomers equaled one-third of our country's entire population during those years.

A few years ago, Ken Dychtwalk, PhD, stated, "As teenagers, boomers bought 43 percent of records sold, 53 percent of movie tickets, and 55 percent of sodas. Four years later, the colleges were overwhelmed by the number of people enrolling. Ten years later, the housing market was stunned by the number of people buying first homes. The first of the boomers are now turning 50 plus. Every eight seconds one of them is receiving an invitation from the American Association of Retired Persons."[1]

The majority of baby boomers will turn 65 between the years 2010 and 2030. As this generation enters that stage in life, you can bank on the fact that they are not going to just roll over and die, but will fight every inch of the way to retain the youthfulness they remember so well.

How will baby boomers deal with aging? Maybe you are a baby boomer—how are you dealing with aging? Author Jeff Ostroff exposes the heartbeat of the boomer generation: "Having built their identity as America's youth generation, the boomers will not enter the second 50 years of life with a whimper. Instead, they'll do everything they can to delay or counteract the effects of aging."[2]

This aging generation, along with the growing numbers in the senior marketplace, is not accepting the over-the-hill mentality. Instead, they are changing the meaning of fitness. The baby boom market is predicted to have tremendous growth over the next decades, especially in the healthcare and fitness service areas. That's because fighting the aging process has become the number one target for this huge section of our population. Those who once possessed the curvaceous figures and Adonis-like bodies will not submit to the aging process without a fight. They will not give in to the mentality that life is over after 40.

With the greater percentage of boomers turning 50, older adults are now the fastest-growing segment in the U.S. population today.[3] According to the United Nations Population Division, this age wave is expected to continue well into the middle of this century.[4]

In 1900, there were about 75.9 million Americans. At the end of 1999, there were 75.9 million Americans over the age of 50.[5]

I have always envisioned being around in the mid-21st century. I think it would be extraordinary to tell stories to the young 50-year-old fitness enthusiasts at the gym then. Watching their expressions will be priceless when I tell them about living back in the medieval days, when television came only in black and white. But I want to be in good health when I talk to them. Dr. Robert Butter, CEO of the International Longevity Center, states, "While ideas about aging are improving, Americans still need to do a better job of preparing for old age."[6]

Today, approximately 80 percent of older Americans reportedly suffer from some form of chronic back pain.[7] Millions experience the day-to-day nagging pain of arthritis in the knees, hips, and hands. Then there are the ones who have RA (rheumatoid arthritis) a systemic autoimmune condition. Many have orthopedic conditions as well as other ailments.

Yet living longer and healthier is the forecast for the boomers. Most are expecting to go through their later years more youthfully than the previous generation did because they will work harder at it. I'm not suggesting that we will not experience pain or discomfort in our aging years, but to be crippled because of lack of effort or laziness is our own fault. I have always said that I would rather check out of life at 90 miles per hour than be forced to use a walker for the last twenty years due to neglecting and abusing my body.

I don't presume my tomorrows are guaranteed. So I am of the belief that if people make regular exercise, eating foods compatible to their blood type, and dietary supplements a constant part of their lives, they will live longer and if not longer, healthier. There's an article in the newspaper or online almost daily giving evidence that we can increase our life spans by doing these things.

As we age, we all should have the desire to create a greater quality of life for ourselves and our loved ones. When your health is upside down, everything you have going on in your life comes to a screeching halt!

||||||||||||||||||||||||| HEALTHY TIP |||||||||||||||||||||||||

The aging process actually begins when a person is in his or her twenties and thirties. Most people soar through their next 10 to 20 years either ignoring or being unaware of the fact that their bodies are aging. Then they reach their 40s, when many of the anti-aging hormones drop off significantly. Finally, when people reach their 50s and 60s, they indeed start feeling and seeing the effects of natural aging.

IS DETERIORATION INEVITABLE?

Pain in the joints—knees, ankles, hips, shoulders, elbows, and spine—is a malady associated with aging. The joints are connected and attached with soft tissue, referred to as ligaments and tendons, which connect the bone to muscle and muscle to muscle. Unfortunately, our joints can undergo some severe damage and destruction from falls, accidents, sports-related injuries—or just from the aging process itself.

Back in the day some 30 years ago, I put my body and joints through some very vigorous and strenuous training sessions as a competitive power lifter. From slipping on a platform in an attempt to dead lift 700 pounds to the 650 pound barbell on my shoulder burying me straight down to floor, it's no wonder today I am dealing with deteriorating hip and back joints. But my condition is sports-related and may be totally different from yours.

When we look back at the accidents, falls, and chronic illnesses we may have experienced in life plus what our bodies go through just in the natural course of aging, it is imperative to learn what to do to slow down the deteriorating effects of aging, so as we continue in life we can maintain as much good quality years as possible.

With time and overuse, the cartilage in a joint starts to degenerate, and the joint may be rubbing bone against bone instead of being protected by the soft cartilage. Consequently, the joints can become painful and inflamed from cartilage degeneration as well as osteoporosis and arthritis.

The sad reality is that as people age, they become less physically active. They sit more, drive instead of walk, take the escalator instead of the stairs, and do less than they did when they were younger. This lack of activity actually contributes to the joint problem, lessening the chance of having healthy joints and making old age painful.

On the other hand, sometimes pain causes the lack of activity. As the human body ages, the joints naturally begin to wear down. Then pain sets in, which causes lifestyle limitations and sometimes disabilities. Because the pain is so great, the individual ceases doing much in the way of activities; consequently, arthritic-like inflammation sets in, which immobilizes and cripples.

That seems to paint a dim picture of aging, but the good news is we can take some preventative and protective measures to strengthen those joints and keep them stable, strong, and pain-free.

Today, continued research and discoveries point to the idea that the aging process can be prevented and in some cases reversed. Cells can be revitalized and we can regain some of our youth. But is longevity itself our goal? I believe our goal should be to live as healthy as possible by preserving and protecting our body regardless of how old we are.

It has become common for aging people to suffer from heart attacks, high blood pressure, strokes, cancer, arthritis, Alzheimer's, and degenerative diseases. These conditions account for approximately 90 percent of the natural aging process.[8] So it is difficult to imagine that these illnesses might actually be symptoms of something greater taking place.

If we are willing to change our thinking, to quit accepting as gospel the idea that because we are aging we automatically should be suffering, then we have a good chance of living longer with a greater quality of life. It is now thought possible for a person to live to be 100 or more and still be healthy and full of vitality.

Knowledge is the key to success, and application of it is the power.

What does the baby-boomer generation want as they enter the fall and winter of their lives? They want to feel good and maintain their youthful appearance, and they are prepared to fight the aging process every step of the way. What they are looking for is quality of life!

The war is on and the battle trumpet has sounded. Let's join the huge segment of today's population who is fighting the aging process.

CHRONOLOGICAL AGE

When are people considered older adults? Physically, studies show that when people enter their sixth decade, they start losing muscular strength, size, and function.[9] The U.S. Census Bureau defines seniors as persons 65 and older, while many businesses offer discounts for people 55 and older. The American Association of Retired Persons considers anyone 50 years of age a senior citizen. In fact, when I turned 50, I received a gold award checking account from my bank. I guess we have to take 'em where we can get 'em, eh?

America's senior population is getting older all the time. The 65 to 74 age group is eight times larger today than it was in 1900, while the 75 to 84 age group is 16 times larger. The over-85 age group is 31 times larger.[10] The female population is outgrowing the male population. For example, the average ratio is 143 senior women to every 100 senior men.

As age increases, the ratios widen. While there are 119 women to every 100 men at ages 65 to 69, the number increases to 248 to 100 over age 85.[11]

Chronological age is valuable to consider. Though we cannot stop the clock on the wall we also can't evaluate the aging process solely by chronological age; it has limitations. That's why we have to also consider functional age.

FUNCTIONAL AGE

Have you ever seen a 65-year-old man or woman running in a marathon? It's more and more common these days. Then there's the 65-year-old you often help put his groceries in the car because it's a struggle for him. Both of these people are age 65, yet their functional ages are vastly different.

There is nothing we can do to change our chronological age. Our history on this earth comprises exactly the number of years from the day we were born until today. But as we have observed, chronological age is not an accurate monitoring device to determine a person's true physical condition. The truer measurement of age is what gerontologists call "functional age."

Functional age is determined by looking at the aging-related or disease-related changes that take place in the body and measuring their effects on daily tasks. Heredity, gender, physical injuries, lifestyle, and chronic diseases all affect a person's functional age.

An active 70-year-old who is aging gracefully can have the functional age of a 60-year-old. On the other hand, a 70-year-old person who has been hampered with illness or multiple medical problems may have the functional age of an 80-year-old.

Functional age is also affected by the attitude of the aging adults. People who hit the age of 40 are told they are over the hill. We have to be careful not to accept this idea, even subconsciously, because it can cause our state of mind to do just that: go downhill. We can now stay youthful and live a life free of diseases well into our later years, so our chronological age has loosened its once strong hold on us.

It has been my experience that as people reach midlife and start taking care of their bodies and their health, they not only begin functioning physically as they did when they were younger, but they also develop the more youthful and vibrant mental attitude that goes along with it.

I have always said that if people would make regular exercise, food selections for their blood type, and proper dietary supplements part of their everyday lives, they would have to think hard when asked how old they are. Reports have suggested that men and women who are athletically and nutritionally fit can actually function as many as 10 to 20 years younger than their chronological age.

Let me give you an example.

My wife, Lori, and I went out for dinner one evening with an older couple who were friends of Lori's. During dinner the husband shared with me how he loves to exercise. Three days a week he drives to the YMCA and does 30 minutes of swimming, 45 minutes of water aerobics and then attends a 45-minute aerobic class in the gym. He said he has never felt better in life. His mind is sharp, he takes his supplements daily, and he has lots of energy. He is thrilled that he started exercising 15 years ago.

When he said that, I did some quick mental calculations. I knew he was 90 years young. That meant this little Hercules sitting across from me had started all that exercising when he was 75! His functional age was certainly quite a bit lower than his chronological age.

That's the goal—getting our functional age as low as possible. Those who exercise have a lower functional age than those who do not. Plus, after the age of 25, the sedentary person loses approximately one-half pound of muscle per year. By the age of 70, about 40 percent of muscle mass is lost if muscle activation or stimulation is not applied.[12]

SENIOR FUNCTIONAL CLASSIFICATIONS

To determine age by functional capacity, a functional classification has been developed.[13]

Physically elite. This group represents a very small percentage of seniors. They train on a daily basis and compete in sports such as the

Senior Olympics or triathlons. Or they participate regularly in vigorous activities or group fitness classes. These seniors can participate in high-risk activities like weightlifting and usually perform at the highest level.

Physically fit. This is a larger group than the elite group, but it is still a small percentage of the population. These seniors typically participate in exercise sessions at least two times per week. They venture out and participate in sports such as tennis. They are capable of participating in endurance sports like power walking, and they are at low risk for falling into the "physically frail" category.

Physically independent. This group of seniors shows signs of loss in balance, coordination, strength, and flexibility. They are the largest group of seniors and range from fairly active to somewhat functionally independent. They may engage in crafts or gardening and perhaps take light walks. They participate in low-level activities such as playing golf. They don't show any debilitating symptoms, but an injury or illness could affect their mobility and physical function. They are apt to fall into the "physically frail" category.

Physically frail. These seniors perform daily activities that are not very demanding, such as shopping and cleaning. They are capable of light activities, but usually sit around and watch television. In many cases, they just stay at home.

Physically dependent. This group represents a small percentage of seniors who are often in wheelchairs and need home care. Basically, they spend much of their money on healthcare.

Totally disabled. This small group of seniors cannot stand or walk. They must rely on complete assistance from professional healthcare staff.

Reading these categories is sobering, isn't it? Please don't lose hope, whether you have chronic pain and aren't able to exercise much or are just full of aches and pain, let's find out how we can fight the aging process.

RENEWING YOUR MIND

- Stay physically active!

- Your functional age can be younger than your chronological age.

- Reduce pain and stress by exercising every day.

- Strengthening your muscles will help support your joints and prevent or reduce arthritic pain.

CHAPTER 34

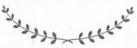

EXERCISE: THE ANTI-AGING SILVER BULLET

"The closest thing to the anti-aging pill is exercise,"
—DR. ALEX LEIF, Harvard Medical School.[1]

Regular physical activity can help the body maintain, repair, and improve itself. Older people, even those who are disabled or ill, can and should take part in some form of exercise program. Exercise strengthens the heart and lungs, lowers blood pressure, and protects against the onset of adult diabetes. It builds, tones, and strengthens muscles and keeps the joints and tendons more flexible. Physical activity gives people more energy, lessens tension and anxiety, and also improves sleep. All in all, exercise contributes to longevity.

Research shows that exercise is an important key component for preventing and treating heart disease, osteoporosis, frailty, diabetes, obesity, and depression. Exercise can be an effective weapon in the fight against these diseases. Exercise will also help you rebound after sickness or illness and injury quicker than if you remain sedentary.

HEALTHY TIP

Fighting Osteoporosis

Exercise can strengthen bones, thereby slowing down the process of osteoporosis. Exercising 30 to 60 minutes three times weekly can help fight osteoporosis.

Fighting Coronary Heart Disease

A combination of strength training and aerobic training will increase the strength and efficiency of the heart muscles. A strong heart eases the workload. If the heart doesn't have to work as hard, it will probably last longer.

Fighting Noninsulin-Dependent Diabetes

The body's ability to use glucose slows down with age. Exercise is a natural preventative that may increase insulin sensitivity, which helps keep blood glucose levels under control for the long haul.

Fighting Obesity

Body weight is best controlled with the combination of proper diet and regular exercise. An individual who is obese and physically inactive must be selective in choosing an exercise program. Even walking can be difficult, so a gradual but consistent approach should be applied.

Fighting Frailty

Frailty in older people can be reversed with regular exercise. People in their mid-80s to mid-90s who exercise and strengthen their muscles experience more stability and endurance.

Fighting Poor Mental Health

Exercise has been shown to improve a person's self-image and provide a way to vent built-up anxieties, tensions, depression, and fears.

NOT PAIN, BUT GAIN

This maturing generation of boomers is becoming a fitness-conscious people, but they are not interested in the no-pain, no-gain mentality. They are striving for a low-impact to no-impact type of exercising. The boomer is looking for a workout that will save the joints and at the same time produce high energy. The focus is on a better quality of life.

Even though I am a former national competitive power lifter and bodybuilder, I no longer care to compete with the "big boys" at the gym. These days, I am pleased to measure up to my own standards for an energetic and disease-free life that allows me to enjoy life with Lori and accommodate my family—including my grandchildren. It is important to me that "Papa Joe" be a picture of vitality and health that exudes discipline and dedication rather than some withered-away fixture that my grandkids see every Sunday afternoon sunken into the easy chair because I gave up on life or had a negative attitude.

So, fitness for the boomer is growing more diverse. As the search for social fulfillment in the later years grows, so do the fitness options. These options include over-50 sports leagues and group activities, such as tennis, golfing, bowling, water aerobics; walking and bicycling should become a continuing part of the aging boomer's life.

Cardiovascular workouts are absolutely necessary for burning unwanted layers of fat and keeping the ticker healthy. It is estimated that nearly five million people a year are diagnosed with coronary heart disease.[2] The prevention of this disease and the maintenance of a healthy body weight requires incorporating a form of regular cardiovascular exercise either daily or every other day. My suggestion—and the Surgeon General's suggestion—is 30 minutes a day of exercise.

Exercises that target balance and coordination, motor flexibility, and improvement in posture are more important after age 50. Water workouts are very effective for obtaining these improvements. When I was having prolotherapy treatments on my pelvis ligaments and tendons,

I spent many months in my swimming pool doing water workouts to prevent atrophy (weakening of muscles) and strengthening them without the concern of gravity and pressure on my hip and lower back joints.

Strength training is now more recognized than ever for its positive impact on retaining strong, healthy muscles. It's amazing that as people age, some are fortunate enough to dodge the heart attack bullet, only to die from a fall. Physicians and sports medicine report that 40 percent of adults over the age of 65 fall at least once a year.[3] Subsequently, strength training is becoming a part of the boomers' workouts.

Strength training, also called resistance training, is no longer limited just to the bodybuilder. In fact, everyone can benefit from strength training. The American College of Sports Medicine places more emphasis on strength training than any other type, incorporating it in aerobic training for a well-rounded training program.

Since the late 1990s and early 2000 there has been a shift in emphasis from cardiovascular training to strength training. Traditionally, medical experts have focused much of their attention on cardiovascular training for improved health and reduction in heart disease. But these older guidelines ignored the musculoskeletal system.

Problems associated with the musculoskeletal system create a new concern for aging adults who want to keep their functional independence. For instance, as people age, their bodies become more fragile because activity levels decrease. This is compounded by a loss in bone and muscle mass. If we do not use our bodies, we will lose them! For many people, the problem isn't aging—it's disuse. Barry Franklin, PhD, president of the American College of Sports Medicine, states, "People who don't exercise regularly suffer a 1 percent loss in aerobic fitness every year starting at age 20. But that loss can be restored years later through three months of steady walking, jogging or biking."[4]

Today the YMCA workout rooms and even some of the gyms are graced with people in their 70s, 80s, and 90s. *Modern Maturity* reports, "Whether chasing gold medals or running around the neighborhood, 50-plus America is on the move. More and more people are toning up, slimming down, and attaining a fitness level belying their years."[5]

Many health professionals today are agreeing that strength training might actually be preferred over aerobic training and other activities as the most effective means of countering the aging process. As we live longer and face the challenges of aging, I believe strength training is going to be the key that will help seniors improve their health, functional capacities, quality of life, and independent lifestyle.

I find it to be true that older adults who are exercising regularly and doing strength training as a major part of their routine are surpassing all their peers in their sports and recreational activities. And their physical activity and fitness level carries over to a positive mental attitude. Strength training provides so many benefits that it should be part of your strategy if you desire a better quality of life through your later years—and who doesn't?

Six Benefits of Strength Training

- *Metabolism increases and body composition changes.* With strength training, the body burns calories more efficiently. As people develop additional muscle mass, their basal metabolic rate (BMR), or the body's ability to burn more calories at rest, increases. This helps maintain a healthy weight. Plus, with strength training, people have more muscle mass and less fat. Strength training overcomes sarcopenia, or muscle loss.

- *Functional ability grows.* Strength training makes everyday tasks easier and helps people keep their independence. Arthritic-like pain and disability lessens. Strength training strengthens joints and increases joint lubrication and stability, a pure natural way to overcome painful and weak joints.

- *Bones become stronger.* Strength training fights osteoporosis by increasing bone mineral density. The increased strength of bones, muscles, and connective tissue causes a decrease in the risk of injury.

- *Healthier mind.* Strength training improves mental alertness and self-worth, which fights depression—a condition that has become more and more common among our seniors.

- *Insulin sensitivity improves.* Strength training improves insulin sensitivity and glucose regulation, which stabilizes blood sugar. This contributes to a steady energy level.

- *A greater quality of life and extended functional independence is experienced.* As a general rule, people who maintain their physical strength are able to perform everyday activities and tasks much easier and well past the traditional retirement timeframe.

HELPING THE JOINTS

If you are the typical mature adult or aging boomer, you are probably experiencing joint pain. The two worst things you can do for your joints: medication and living a sedentary life. I have counseled many older clients who end up having stomach disorders from taking anti-inflammatory medication chronically for their arthritic pain. The problem then becomes twofold: stomach problems in addition to joint pain.

|||||||||||||||||||||||||||| **HEALTHY TIP** ||||||||||||||||||||||||||||

The Benefits of Strength Training

- Metabolism increases and body composition changes.
- Functional ability grows.
- Arthritic-like pain and disability lessens.
- Bones become stronger.
- The mind becomes healthier and more positive.
- Insulin sensitivity improves.
- Improved quality of life.

- Extended functional independence.

||||||||||||||||||||||||||||||||||||||||||||||||||||||||||||||||||||||||||||||||||||||||||||||||||||||||||||||||||

It's a catch-22. Due to high level of pain older clients think they cannot do much of anything; consequently they are less active—living sedentary lives. Their condition cannot improve because of inactivity, and they lose that good quality of life they once knew. When people are inactive, their muscles atrophy, or weaken in size and strength. Consequently, all the strain and pressure is directly on the joint. So strengthening the muscles and soft tissue that support the joint is part of the plan to rebuild and strengthen the joints.

Here are some preventative and protective measures to take:

- *Exercise* strengthens muscles, ligaments, and tendons, which directly support the joints which in turn takes pressure off the joints and reduces your level of pain. Exercise the major muscle groups—legs, back, chest, shoulders, core (abs), and arms. Exercise each muscle group two to three times per week. Perform eight to ten repetitions for three sets per exercise. You can utilize free weights or weight machines, as well as flexible stretch cords or bands. NOTE: exercise selection should be determined by your current physical condition!

- *Use fitness balls.* I have experienced over and over one of the best methods for strengthening all 27 stabilizer muscles—using a fitness ball. You see them in the YMCA and other fitness facilities. Exercising with a fitness ball requires your body to use stabilizer muscles to keep you on the ball. In return, you become more stable in walking, jogging, dancing; if you golf, you will notice much more balance and control of your swing.

- *Crunches,* not sit-ups, are excellent exercises for strengthening the stomach muscles or abs, which are part of the core muscles and do not require any particular piece of equipment. As you strengthen the abdominal muscles, you indirectly make your lower back healthier, stronger, and pain-free. A strong abdominal wall also stabilizes the movements of your upper torso or trunk.

- *Stretching* is necessary for developing and increasing range of motion (ROM) around the joints. Joints become stiff, sore, and short-range when they are not active and not stretched. Increasing the ROM increases blood circulation, keeps the joint lubricated, enhances everyday tasks, helps prevent muscle injuries, and makes enjoying life with exciting activities more likely.

- *Static stretching* is recommended because it is a gentle form of stretching. Stretch the legs, arms, or back to the point where the muscles feel comfortably tight. Hold that position for at least 15 seconds, then return to a relaxed position. Repeat this stretching technique two to three times. Be sure to breathe freely. Do not hold your breath. The idea is to relax your body so the muscles will elongate and open the range of motion of the joint. Stretching can be done daily, especially after exercising.

STARTING AN ANTI-AGING EXERCISE PROGRAM

If you are under 35 years of age and in good health, you probably don't need to see a doctor before beginning your exercise program. But if you are over 35 and have been inactive for several years, you should consult your physician first. At any age, if you have or have had high blood pressure, dizzy spells, arthritis, heart trouble, ligament or tendon problems, or a family history of heart attacks, then you should consult your doctor before beginning your program.

If you are planning to embark on a strength training program but are not quite sure where to begin, let me give you a few suggestions:

Interview personal trainers at your local YMCA or health clubs. Get references from people you trust. Ask them to do an evaluation of your exercise history, medical history, goals, and likes and dislikes pertaining to exercise. Then discuss which activities or exercises will best suit your interests and genetics or body types. The more accurate your exercise selections are based on your genetic structure plus your favorite exercises, the greater the likelihood of success.

If you go it alone try the following: Start out by performing two sets of 8 to 12 repetitions for basic strength building of the major muscle groups—thighs, back, chest, shoulders, arms, and abdominals. The amount of weight or resistance you select should be enough to feel challenging by the end of each set. When you perform each exercise, never hold your breath, simply breathe as freely as you can. Full range of motion throughout each exercise provides a complete stimulus per muscle trained. If the last set of an exercise is completed with ease, that's your indication to move up in the weight or resistance. Usually a 5 to 10 pound increase will suffice.

Your level of fitness dictates how much to do under all circumstances. If you try to do too much at the beginning, you will simply slow down your progress.

Have fun with it. Mix it up. Do some weights one week, then some machines another. Be sure to throw in some recreational activities outside the gym such as tennis, volleyball, golf, or any sport or activity that will keep the blood flowing.

RENEWING YOUR MIND

- Be creative with exercise—include the family.
- Set goals that are attainable.
- Challenge yourself.

- Seek the help of a fitness professional who can adjust your exercise to meet your specific requirement: joint pain, arthritis, age, current condition.

- Always listen to your body.

- Walk away from every workout like you could have done more.

- Stay hydrated during workouts.

- Exercise with purpose: improve posture, rehabilitate after injury, weight loss, etc.

CHAPTER 35

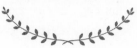

SUPPLEMENTS

"Food is your baseline for nutrition and nutritional
supplements fill the gaps!" —Dr. Joe

I have always been a firm believer that if someone continues to treat the symptoms and ignore the root problem, there can only be one result: a lesser quality of life. Addressing only the symptoms (whether health-related, emotional, or spiritual) will cause a person to die prematurely.

If your house were on fire, you would call the fire department. When they arrived, would you prefer that the firefighters hose down the gushing smoke or the fire itself? I hope your answer is the fire!

Medicating or fighting symptoms after they appear is not the answer. Regular exercise, eating foods compatible with your blood type, and dietary supplementation are the keys for healthy longevity. Hormonal control and balance are also necessary for both men and women for a good quality of life.

HORMONES AND AGING

Hormones regulate and influence the functions of the body. As we grow older, our hormone production diminishes, thus causing the appearance of aging. Our bodies lose some of the ability to function as they did when we were young. But we do have the resources that help to prevent this. Aging boomers in search of a more youthful and vibrant entrance into their later years can take supplemental hormones in addition to exercising regularly, eating instinctively for their blood type and taking dietary supplements in general.

The key to slowing down and possibly turning around the symptoms that identify the over-the-hill gang is to bring the body's hormone production back to its normal levels. Age-related diseases, such as heart disease, arthritis, high blood pressure, elevated cholesterol, and loss of skin elasticity can be prevented or slowed down by natural hormonal therapy.

The hormones we tend to need as we age are DHEA or (dehydroepiandrosterone), estrogen, testosterone, progesterone, thyroid, insulin, pregnenolone, and human growth hormone (HGH)[1] These hormones are all interrelated and must work in harmony to create the synergistic effect required to prevent aging. Of course there are plenty more like cortisol, adrenalin, glucagons, etc. The key is to establish homeostasis or a balance between them. With a simple saliva test or blood draw ordered by your physician or naturopathic doctor and some periodical monitoring, you can establish and maintain a hormonal balance in your body.

Aging boomers can improve their health and decrease potential illnesses associated with the aging process by taking supplements to boost their anabolic hormone levels. The question is, when does a person start? That question reminds me of people trying to decide when to get a face-lift. Do they wait until their skin is hanging down to their chest, or do they catch it in the earlier stages? Do you start using HGH or DHEA when you're 80, or do you start when you're 50 years of age? With a visit to see your physician, maybe your best shot at a fountain of youth is right around the corner.

DHEA

Several years ago I made an appointment with a doctor friend of mine to have some blood work done. I wanted to know my blood lipids and my DHEA sulfate levels. I felt good, but work was starting to cause me to drag. I assumed my counts would be normal, but I wanted to check just in case.

The test results indicated that my level of DHEA sulfate was actually below the low-normal range. That puzzled the doctor and me because typically when a person takes care of his health as I do, most readings show up in the normal ranges. After discussing my business schedule and the demands on my time, the doctor and I agreed that the low reading was most likely associated with stress in my life.

So he wrote a prescription for DHEA. I started taking it orally and I experienced an improved state of general well-being. I felt somewhat stronger and showed better responses to my training. After one month I went back for another DHEA sulfate test, and this time my level was in the normal range.

It is important to have your DHEA sulfate levels checked through blood testing. DHEA plays a tremendous role in balancing your hormones. This precursor hormone, normally produced in the adrenal glands, is like the conductor of a symphony. It directs the secretions of certain glands to meet the hormonal demands of your body.

When you were in your early 20s, your body had higher levels of DHEA. But as the aging process continued, those levels started to plummet. Though your body was manufacturing 30 milligrams of DHEA at age 20, unfortunately by age 60, it only drums up about 5 milligrams.[2] A reduction in your body's DHEA contributes to diseases associated with getting old.

"When blood levels of DHEA are increased to the level one had at a younger age, many diseases just melt away. The body seems to be fully capable of using supplemental DHEA as if it were processed in the body," says Dr. Julian Whitaker.[3]

By keeping your DHEA levels up to their maximum, you will help your body be better fit to fight against heart disease, cancers, cardiovascular diseases, and obesity. Plus, normal levels will assist in creating a hormonal balance among all the hormones listed earlier.

HUMAN GROWTH HORMONE (HGH)

The increased levels of these major hormones (promoted by normal levels of DHEA) promote the human growth hormone (HGH) production. Human growth hormone is a protein produced in the pituitary gland that stimulates the liver to produce somatomedins, which stimulate growth of bone and muscle. The production of this hormone peaks during adolescence, then steadily declines with age.[4]

HGH levels are at about 400 as a teenager. But when you arrive at the ripe age of 70, they are way down to 100.[5] Ask your physician for an IGF-1 (insulin-like growth factor) test. Determining your IGF-1 (insulin-like growth factors) levels is a way to monitor your HGH levels. An HGH dietary supplement in pill form is available. But it is ideal to work with your physician to see if you should get on a program of daily injectable HGH.

OTHER LEVELS TO MONITOR

Because the lowered production of hormones that comes with age has a link to improper fat metabolization, having blood lipids tests taken every 18 months or so is a good idea. This is to monitor your cholesterol levels, the HDL (good cholesterol) and LDL (bad cholesterol) in your blood.

||||||||||||||||||||||||||||| **HEALTHY TIP** |||||||||||||||||||||||||||||

Potential Benefits of HGH Therapy

- Improved memory
- Improvement of Alzheimer's disease
- Regeneration of the brain, liver, and other organs
- Improved sexual function
- Enhanced immunity with increased resistance to infection
- Improved healing of wounds and fractures
- Hair regrowth and color restored

- Improved vision
- Improved exercise tolerance
- Increased muscle mass
- Reduction of fat and cellulite
- Increased energy and stamina
- Increase in HDL (good cholesterol) and decrease in LDL (bad cholesterol)
- Reversal of osteoporosis and strengthening of bones
- Elevation of moods
- Improved sleep patterns
- Improved elasticity and thickness of skin[6]

It is also important to monitor levels of homocysteine, an important amino acid used for building particular body proteins. Too high a level of homocysteine can have a damaging effect on arteries, causing arteriosclerosis and possibly leading to heart attacks and strokes. Some people, regardless of diet, are prone to high levels of homocysteine, which must be controlled.

Your level should not exceed ten, and ideally it should be around seven to eight. Certain B vitamins control homocysteine levels, particularly B6. This is a water-soluble supplement, so I suggest taking the Recommended Daily Allowance.

ANTIOXIDANTS

Many individuals suffer from pain and illnesses caused by impaired and unbalanced molecules called free radicals. Superoxides, hydroxyl radicals, peroxides, and hydroperoxides are examples of free radicals. These impaired molecules attach themselves to healthy cells in the body of the host.

They are not proud invaders; they will settle anywhere. Wherever they attach themselves, they cause a rapid oxidation process, which results in cell damage. If there is free-radical damage to the cells in the walls of the arteries, then plaque buildup is imminent. If cellular damage occurs in the joints due to these culprits, then arthritic pain and discomfort can follow.

Thousands upon thousands of free radicals enter your body every time you inhale the fumes from automobiles, buses, and planes. They also affect us when we exercise because we oxidize our cells then. If you think you can escape them by not going outside or exercising, guess again. Free-radical damage occurs from breathing itself. (Do I have to mention what you would have to do to avoid these guys completely?)

By now almost everyone has heard of antioxidants. These nutrient substances function as scavengers, neutralizing the free-radical molecules. They oppose oxidation and inhibit reactions promoted by oxidation. For example, if there is damage to the lining of the cells in the arterial wall, the antioxidant neutralizes the oxidation action that is destroying the cells and stops the damage. The cells that have not been destroyed can be strengthened by the antioxidant.

Because it is impossible to avoid the attacks of these free radicals, the best thing to do is to defend against them. If you can neutralize their destructive forces and strengthen some of your cells that have been weakened, then you are doing about all you can.

Some antioxidants that can be taken as dietary supplements are vitamin A, vitamin E, selenium, beta carotene, coenzyme Q10, zinc and green tea. Super antioxidants that range from 20 to 50 times the potency of vitamins C and E are called proanthocyanidins. They are generally extracted from the grape seed and are very potent, yet nontoxic.

All antioxidants contribute to strengthening the heart muscles, cleaning the arteries, fighting against cholesterol and cancer, and reducing swelling from arthritic pain.

Do your best to avoid the activities that contribute to free-radical damage.

START FIGHTING THE AGING PROCESS TODAY

All this information on beating aging might sound too good to be true, but the reality is that many health-conscious people today are already enjoying the benefits of making healthier lifestyle changes as they enter the later years of their lives.

|||||||||||||||||||||||||||||||**HEALTHY TIP**|||||||||||||||||||||||||||||

Here are a few other measures you can take to avoid some of the problems associated with free radicals:

- Quit smoking.
- Avoid unsaturated oils, especially the rancid oils often used to deep-fry foods at fast-food restaurants.
- Avoid toxic chemicals, fumes from cars and trucks.
- Avoid food additives such as nitrites and nitrates.
- Avoid exposure to X-rays and radiation.

In order for your body to continue to function healthfully and energetically, it requires maintenance. The sooner you decide to start giving your body that attention, the sooner you will reap the benefits—more energy, less sickness, less pain, more mental alertness, more disease-free living, better mobility, fewer doctor bills, more fun, and a greater quality of life. It is difficult to break old habits and make new adjustments, but focusing on the end results will keep you on track.

Chronological age does not have to interfere so greatly with the quality of your life. Aging adults are becoming more and more aware of the health benefits that come from living an active lifestyle. Subsequently, their chronological age is no longer a factor, limiting them to the premature use of walkers and wheelchairs. Instead, they find themselves experiencing the youthful and energetic lifestyle they did in years prior.

Learning a little more about how your body functions and what it requires to function as it did when you were younger will help you make these lifestyle changes easier. As you begin experiencing the benefits from healthy lifestyle practices, your entire life takes on a whole new level of wellness, then you will appreciate how wonderfully your body has been fashioned. Then your hope for a healthier and more youthful life as you get older will become a reality.

As you apply many of these healthy tips and lifestyle changes, you begin to have a greater appreciation for life. It is going to be small changes over a long period of time that will bring lasting results. Whether you are struggling with chronic pain, recent injuries, or overall weakness and disease, please know that your body will heal itself. Instead of following the conventional medical methods of treating your symptoms as the first line of defense, give your body the benefit of the doubt and test everything natural, first!

Totally exhaust every natural alternative protocol, modality, treatment, remedy, etc. that's available to you. Allow natural health to be your first line of defense for eradicating the root cause of your painful symptoms or poor health condition. Only when all else has failed, then you may have no choice but to seek conventional medicine and its approach to dealing with your symptoms.

RENEWING YOUR MIND

- Eat according to your blood type and exercise regularly to prevent endocrine system disorders.

- Avoid prolonged stress. When stress becomes overwhelming, it can cause hormone dysfunction, weaken your immune system, and make you susceptible to infection.

- Reach your ideal weight and keep it. This is a great prevention measure for defending yourself from type II diabetes, an endocrine problem.

- Get your hormone levels checked. A saliva test or blood draw will show your current levels.

- Take proper nutritional supplementation for your hormones.

- Stay physically active with regular exercise and recreational activities.

- Keep a youthful mind; think healthy and positive thoughts.

- Learn to laugh more; enjoy life and those who you love.

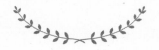

CONCLUSION

Life does not always give us options to choose from when physical trauma, sickness, disease, and injuries befall us. And because we tend to function out of habit, it takes discipline to make the changes that will benefit us currently and into our future. Healthy lifestyle changes, step by step, provide a solid foundation that allows our state of mind and physical condition to fall into balance and harmony with the way we were intended to function.

The wisdom behind healthy lifestyle practices whether from exercise, nutritional supplements, positive thinking, proper sleep and rest, goes well beyond biceps and waistlines. It has to do with building a body (and mental fortitude) that is resilient and durable so that when the storms of life hit (and they will) you can rebound, recover, and lift yourself back to good health in the shortest time possible.

As you walk through your healing day by day you will discover the way to live beyond your chronic pain by open-mindedness and willingness to test everything. As you realize you are not alone in this painful season and believe there is a life that is pain-free that awaits you, it's just a matter of time until you experience a new healthy and vibrant life.

Live in peace!

ENDNOTES

INTRODUCTION

1. Global Industry Analysts, Inc., "Pain Management: A Global Strategic Business Report," Vocus/PRWEB, (January 10, 2011),; http://www.prweb.com/releases/2011/1/prweb8052240.htm (accessed 11/13/13).

2. Committee on Advancing Pain Research, Care, and Education: *Relieving Pain in America: A Blueprint for Transforming Prevention, Care, Education, and Research*, The National Academies Press, 2011, 1, http://books.nap.edu/openbook.php?record_id=13172 (accessed 12/13/13).

3. American Diabetes Association, "Statistics About Diabetes," (January 26, 2011), http://diabetes.org/diabetes-basics/statistics (accessed 12/13/13).

4. Veronique Roger et al, "Heart Disease and Stroke Statistics—2011 Update: A Report from the Association," Circulation 123, (2011): 20, http://circ.ahajournals.org/content/123/4/e18.full.pdf (accessed 12/13/13).

5. American Cancer Society, "Prevelance of Cancer: How Many People Have Cancer?" (October 14, 2013), http://www.cancer.org/cancer/cancerbasics/cancer-prevalance (accessed 12/13/13).

CHAPTER 5—DEEP BREATHING TO CONTROL PAIN

1. Mark Liponis, *Ultra-Longevity* (New York: Little, Brown and Company, 2007).

2.   Robert Gorter, and Erik Peper, *Fighting Cancer: A Nontoxic Approach to Treatment* (Berkeley, CA: North Atlantic Books, 2011).

3.   William Sears, with Martha Sears, *Prime-Time Health* (New York: Little, Brown and Company, 2010).

4.   V.A. Pavlov and K.J. Tracey, "The Cholinergic Anti-inflammatory Pathway," *Brain, Behavior, Immunization 6*, (November 19, 2005): 493-9, http://www.ncbi.nlm.nih.gov/pubmed/15922555 (accessed 12/13/13).

5.   R.P. Sloan et al., "RR Interval Variability is Inversely Related to Inflammatory Markers: The CARDIA Study," Molecular Medicine 13, (March-April 2007): 178-84, http://www.ncbi.nlm.nih.gov/pubmed/17592552 (accessed 12/13/13).

6.   Pavlov and Tracey, "The Cholinergic Anti-inflammatory Pathway."

7.   N.D. Theise and R. Harris, "Postmodern Biology: (Adult) (Stem) Cells Are Plastic, Stochastic, Complex, and Uncertain," HEP 174, (2006): 389-408. http://neiltheise.com/pdfs/PostModExpPh.pdf (accessed 12/13/13).

8.   Liponis, *Ultra-Longevity*.

9.   Sears, *Prime-Time Health*.

10.   Gary L. Wenk, *Your Brain on Food* (New York: Oxford Univ. Press, 2010).

CHAPTER 6—TMS

1.   John E. Sarno, *Healing Back Pain: The Mind-Body Connection* (New York: Grand Central Life & Style, 2010), 3.

2.   Ibid., 29-30.

CHAPTER 7—MAP YOUR CHOICES

1.   Peter D. Hart Research Associates, "Americans Talk About Pain: A Survey Among Adults Nationwide," Research America, (August 2003), http://www.researchamerica.org/uploads/poll2003pain.pdf (accessed 12/14/13).

CHAPTER 8—GLOSSARY OF TREATMENTS

1.

CHAPTER 9—MEDICATIONS

1. Leonard Paulozzi, Chistopher Jones, Karin Mack, Rose Rudd, "Vital Signs: Overdoses of Presciption Opoid Pain Relievers—United States, 1999-2008," Morbidity and Mortality Weekly Report 43, (November 4, 2011): 1487-1492, http://www.cdc.gov/mmwr/preview/mmwrhtml/mm6043a4.htm?s_cid=mm6043a4_w (accesses 12/14/13).

CHAPTER 15—YOUR GENETIC CODE AND YOUR HEALTH

1. Joseph Christiano, *Never Go Back* (Body Redesigning, 2007), 204.
2. Ibid.
3. Ibid.
4. Ibid., 210.

CHAPTER 20—ALKALINE ASH-PRODUCING FOODS

1. Joseph Christiano, *My Body, God's Temple* (Trinity Publishing and Marketing Group, 1998, 2004), 89-90.
2. Ibid.
3. Ibid.
4. Ibid.

CHAPTER 21—COLON HEALTH

1. American Cancer Society, "What is Colorectal Cancer?" (July 30, 2013), http://www.cancer.org/cancer/colonandrectumcancer/detailedguide/colorectal-cancer-key-statistics (accessed 12/15/13).
2. http://www.mayoclinic.org/digestive-system/sls-20076373?s=7.
3. Albert Zehr, *Healthy Steps to Maintain or Regain Natural Good Health* (Abundant Health Publishers, 1996), 35.
4. Ibid.
5. Ibid.
6. Ibid., 38.
7. Ibid.

8.   http://www.dmu.edu/medterms/digestive-system/ digestive-system-diseases/.

9.   Zehr, *Healthy Steps to Maintain or Regain Natural Good Health*, 39.

10. Ibid., 41.

11. Ibid.

12. Carlos M. Viana, *Prescriptions from Paradise: Introduction to Biocompatible Medicine* (Healing Spirit Press, 2012), 58.

CHAPTER 22—PARASITIC INFESTATION

1.   Teresa Schumacher and Toni Schumacher Lund, *Cleansing the Body and the Colon for a Happier and Healthier You* (n.p., 1987), 10.

2.   Ibid.

3.   Dolly Katz, *Miami Herald*, quoted in Schumacher and Lund, *Cleansing the Body and the Colon for a Happier and Healthier You*, 10.

4.   Schumacher and Lund, *Cleansing the Body and the Colon for a Happier and Healthier You*, 10.

5.   Ibid., 13.

6.   Ibid., 11.

7.   Ibid., 26.

8.   Ibid., 15.

CHAPTER 24—THE IMMUNE SYSTEM: ARMED FORCES AGAINST INVADERS

1.   Tulane University, "Hematopathology Images: Lymphocytes," http://tulane.edu/som/departments/pathology/training/ hematopathology_images_05.cfm (accessed 12/16/13).

CHAPTER 25—ENEMY INFILTRATORS

1.   Stewart B. Levy, "The Challenge of Antibiotic Resistance," Scientific American, (March 1, 1998), http://www.sciam .com/1998/0398issue/0398Levy.html (accessed 1999).

2.   Lisa Landymore-Lim, *Poisonous Prescriptions* (Subraco, WA, Australia: PODD, 1994).

3.   Zehr, *Healthy Steps to Maintain or Regain Natural Good Health*, 58.

4. "Innovations in Cancer Therapy," Immunotherapy, http://www
    .cancer.org/treatment/treatmentsandsideeffects/treatmenttypes/
    immunotherapy/immunotherapy-types.

CHAPTER 26—MAINTAIN A STRONG IMMUNE SYSTEM

1. Zehr, *Healthy Steps to Maintain or Regain Natural Good Health*, 59.
2. "Fibromyalgia," Aetna InteliHealth, (August 28, 2012), http://
    www.intelihealth.com/article/fibromyalgia?nid=1801 (accessed
    12/16/13).
3. Ibid.

CHAPTER 27—BENEFITS OF EXERCISE

1. Centers for Disease Control and Prevention, Physical Activity and
    Health: A Report of the Surgeon General, 1996, http://www.cdc.
    gov/nccdphp/sgr/pdf/execsumm.pdf (accessed 12/16/13).

CHAPTER 30—THE IMPORTANCE OF R&R

1. AP, "Heavy online use can mean anxiousness," Miami Herald,
    http://www.miamiherald.com/2013/12/14/3817983/ohio-study
    -heavy-online-use-can.htmlhtml (accessed 12/16/13).
2. Leonard Holmes, "Managing Stress: Too Much of a Good Thing?"
    About.com, (November 21, 2003), http://mentalhealth.about.com/
    cs/stressmanagement/a/invertedu.htm (accessed 12/16/13).

CHAPTER 31—PROGRESSIVE RELAXATION

1. Adapted from the *HFI Workbook,* American College of Sports
    and Medicine, and Stress Management Training Program,
    Adelphi University.

CHAPTER 32—A GOOD NIGHT'S REST

1. http://drhoffman.com/article/healthy-sleep-recharging-your
    -batteries-2/.
2. Ibid.
3. Zehr, *Healthy Steps to Maintain or Regain Natural Good Health,* 109.
4. Ibid., 110.

CHAPTER 33—AGING AND DETERIORATION

1.   Ken Dychtwalk, "Baby Boomers Ready to Get Fit," quoted in Lisa Johnson, "Boomers Bloom," *American Fitness,* November/ December 1996, 45.
2.   Jeff Ostroff, "Successful Marketing to the 50+ Consumer," quoted in Lisa Johnson, "Boomers Bloom," *American Fitness* (November/ December 1996):
3.   Terrie Heinrich Rizzo, and Karl Knopf, "Resistance Training for Older Adults," *Health and Fitness Idea Source* (June 1999): 33.
4.   Ibid.
5.   Bill Burkart, "Marketers Must View Boomers through a New Lens," www.neoa.org/news/archives/marketers_view.html.
6.   Ibid.
7.   Lisa Johnson, "Boomers Bloom," *American Fitness* (November/ December 1996): 47.
8.   www.medicine-antiaging.com/test.htm.
9.   Rizzo and Knopf, "Resistance Training for Older Adults."
10.   Ibid.
11.   Ibid.
12.   Ibid.
13.   Ibid., 34.

CHAPTER 34—EXERCISE: THE ANTI-AGING SILVER BULLET

1.   Mark S. Lander, "Turning Back Time with Exercise," *America Online: Bloodtype 2,* copyright © 2000 by iVillage, Inc.
2.   Johnson, "Boomers Bloom," 47.
3.   Ibid., 45.
4.   "Living to the Max," *Modern Maturity,* July/August 1999.
5.   Ibid.

CHAPTER 35—SUPPLEMENTS

1.   M. Cherrier, S. Plymate, S. Mohan et al., "Relationship between testosterone supplementation and insulin-like growth factor-I levels and cognition in healthy older men," Psychoneuroendocrinology 29, (January 2004): 65-82.

2. "Male Hormone Restoration," *LifeExtension.com*, http://www.lef.org/protocols/male_reproductive/male_hormone_restoration_02 htm (accessed January 18, 2014).

3. Ibid.

4. Dictionary.com—http://dictionary.reference.com/browse/growth+hormone.

5. http://www.ncbi.nlm.nih.gov/pmc/articles/PMC1813007/?page=1.

6. "What Is Anti-Aging Medicine?" *Health and Fitness Journal*, (November 11, 2013), http://www.healthfitnessjournal.com/what-is-anti-aging-medicine.

RESOURCES

CONCENTRACE—LIQUID TRACE MINERALS

 CONCENTRACE Liquid Minerals is a purified concentrated mineral source: a (desalinated) product providing mineral balance for more effective electric connections to nerve endings for alertness and body responses. Many arthritics with bone spurs have taken CONCENTRACE with successful results, dissolving abnormal mineral deposit spurs (bone spurs) and increasing energy and alertness. The dosage recommended on the product increases bowel action and eliminates the problem quickly. For more information, visit www.bodyredesigning.com or call 1-800-259-2639.

BLOODTYPES, BODYTYPES, AND YOU

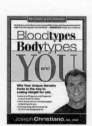 This popular book has been revised and expanded. You will learn how and why to eat foods designed specifically for your blood type—which foods you should eat and which you should avoid. Enjoy 14 varieties of breakfast, lunch, and dinner, plus desserts, snacks, hundreds of recipes, and *more!* Dr. Joe's book explains how your blood type is pivotal in food selection for improving body composition that determines your ability to lose weight and keep it off for life. Discover when eating for your blood type how your body will eliminate painful digestive disorders, gas, bloating, constipation, IBS, and sleepless nights. Also improve your illness profile, lower cholesterol and blood pressure levels, reduce arthritic-like pain, and help stabilize your blood sugar!

"The most accurate and individualized way to eat that improves all areas of your life." —DR. JOE

For more information, visit www.bodyredesigning.com or call 1-800-259-2639.

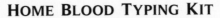

HOME BLOOD TYPING KIT

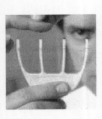

All the materials you need to take one blood type test is in this simple home blood typing kit. Within 15 minutes you can know your blood type. Pretreated mixing card prevents misapplying or cross-contaminating anti-sera. Control panel on mixing card assures reliability. Just read instructions and follow directions for easy testing.

The home blood typing kit comes with: Eldoncard for ABO/Rh, mixing sticks, lancet, alcohol prep, and water pipette. Order one for each family member!

For more information, visit www.bodyredesigning.com or call 1-800-259-2639.

INNER OUT COLON CLEANSING SYSTEM

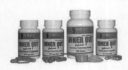

The *Inner Out Colon Cleansing System* is a 14-day, 2-week program designed to generate a progressive cleansing effect on your body in just 14 days. There are three important phases:

Phase 1: Preparation Phase—Prepares the colon. Helps kill off parasites, remove mucus from the colon walls, and may enhance bowel movement.

Phase 2: The Cleansing Phase—The primary colon cleansing and detoxifying effectiveness revolves around the ingredients found in the Phase 2 Cleansing and Detoxifying Powder. These ingredients team together with other nutrients in the capsules to perform a proper colon cleansing and detoxifying process. The clay-like substance has a scrubbing action and a 100:1 absorption power that cleans the wall of the colon and removes toxic buildup and parasites.

Phase 3: The Restoration Phase—Return to eating solids. Take the herbal formula capsules containing probiotics for replenishing good bacteria into your colon.

Cleansing is a great asset in the maintenance of optimum health. Dr. Joe recommends a colon cleanse every 6 months for optimum health.

For more information, visit www.bodyredesigning.com or call 1-800-259-2639.

IMMUNE SUPPORT

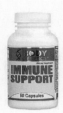

Formulated to help build the immune system naturally! A strong immune system protects you from viruses, germs, parasites, disease, etc. Take daily to keep your immune system strong. The perfect remedy for flu and allergy seasons!

For more information, visit www.bodyredesigning.com or call 1-800-259-2639.

DR. JOE'S PAIN MANAGEMENT NUTRIENTS

Check out Dr. Joe's dietary supplements that are formulated specifically for arthritic-like conditions, inflammation, joint and muscle pain. His NO Pain supplements are pharmaceutical and contain the highest quality of nutrients best suited for relieving pain.

For more information, visit www.bodyredesigning.com or call 1-800-259-2639.

HOME-GROWN BLOOD TYPE VEGETABLE GARDEN PACKAGE

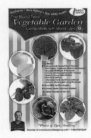

Plant your own home-grown vegetables based on your blood type. No need for acreage to plant huge gardens. This simple and convenient approach to planting your own vegetable seeds makes it possible to grow your garden "in a pot."

All the vegetable seeds are *non*-GMO, Organic, Heirloom and *non-hybrid*.

For more information, visit: www.bloodtypegardens.com or call 1-800-259-2639.

ReJuV U
ADVANCED STEM CELL TECHNOLOGIES
AND HOLISTIC HEALING THERAPIES

For complete information about booking an appointment at Dr. Christiano's ReJuV U clinic, please go to www.re-juv.us or call: 1-800-259-2639. Located at: Sunrise Medical Centre & Hospital East Sunrise Hwy. Freeport, Grand Bahama, Bahamas.

ABOUT THE AUTHOR

In 1978 Joe Christiano opened The York Health Center; in 1985 he opened Body Redesigning by Joseph Christiano. Since then he has helped untold numbers of people prepare and redesign their bodies for competition including correct diet and exercise routines. In the process of training scores of successful men and women, he also helped them recover from injuries by implementing various exercises to strengthen the surrounding muscles and ligaments and prescribed proper diet and nutritional supplements to enhance their recovery.

With his passion to "help people be healthy" and make fitness personal, Body Redesigning's private, one-on-one studios grew to six locations in central Florida. Its clientele base includes top-line executives from Walt Disney World, Universal Studios, Hard Rock Cafe, Planet Hollywood, General Mills, Sea World, plus major law firms, doctors, and Hollywood celebrities such as Bonnie Bedalia, Sylvester Stallone, Michael Bolton, Bryant Levant, plus local TV and radio personalities.

Having been involved in health and fitness both personally and professionally for more than 50 years, he shares a wealth of healthy knowledge to not only competitive individuals but people from all walks of life—no matter what age in life. As a professional fitness trainer/coach consultant he has worked with practically every body type and shape.

He earned a naturopathic doctor degree from Trinity College of Natural Health, which rounded out the years of hands-on, practical experience helping satisfied and healed clients. He also worked hand in hand with medical doctors who had left their mainstream medical practices to become part of alternative medicine where they went from treating symptoms of health disorders to eradicating root causes for total healing.

As an accomplished motivational speaker, life coach, health and wellness expert, Dr. Joe has traveled throughout America, Canada, and the Caribbean empowering people of all ages and walks of life to enrich their lives by addressing the 'whole' person.

If you are interested in Dr. Christiano's coaching services, speaking engagements, TV and radio interviews, please contact Rita at 1-800-259-2639 or rita@bodyredesigning.com.

To contact Dr. Joe directly:

Email: drjoe@bodyredesigning.com

Facebook: Joseph Christiano

Facebook: Body Redesigning

Twitter: @BodyRedesigning

OTHER BOOKS BY JOSEPH CHRISTIANO

Joseph Christiano's Blood Type Diet Series (O, A, B, AB)

Blood Types, Body Types and You

My Body, God's Temple

Seven Pillars of Health

Never Go Back

The Answer is in YOUR Blood Type

Dump the Junk for Parents

Dump the Junk for Kids, K-4 Curriculum